Alkaline Diet

*The Complete Guide for Beginners.
Eat well with Alkaline Diet
Cookbook.*

Delicious Alkaline Recipes

Julene Hearn

Table of Contents

Introduction

Have you been looking for information on the alkaline diet and how it affects the body, but you've yet to find the straightforward information that you want? People who believe in the diet say that replacing acidic foods with alkaline foods will improve your health, fight off diseases, and help you lose weight. However, what about the evidence behind these claims?

Without sounding too technical, the body is constantly working to maintain a healthy pH balance. It likes it when it's a little on the basic or alkaline side. In the following chapters, we will look at what pH is and how it works, but as of right now, the important thing to know is that the scale runs from 0 to 14. Anything over 7 is alkaline and below 7 is acidic.

The Standard American Diet is full of foods that produce acid. It's full of fatty and fried foods, dairy products, red meat, alcohol, refined sugar, and processed carbs. This diet does a lot to the body and very little of it is good. It messes with the liver, kidneys, and the digestive system. This can end up causing health problems like cancer, hypertension, and renal disease.

Nevertheless, if you start filling up your plate with alkaline foods, such as vegetables, beans, leafy greens, fruits, sprouted grains, and more, you will be giving your body a bunch of healthy nutrients and vitamins. Healthy foods will make your cells healthy. A large number of recipes in this book will ensure that you are always satisfied and never bored.

When you get started with the book, you may find that it all seems overwhelming. Don't worry, it is really rather simple. Eating an alkaline diet means that you will choose whole foods and plant-based foods over unhealthy processed foods. There is no need to count calories or remove entire food groups. All you need to do is make sure that you consume more alkaline forming foods than acidic forming foods. You'll be surprised at how quickly you learn what foods you should and shouldn't eat.

The alkaline diet is also perfect for everybody. Also, while it may not have been designed with weight loss in mind, it will help you lose weight. The foods that you do eat will leave you feeling full as well.

It's also a good idea to make sure that you keep up with a regular exercise program, get plenty of sleep, hydrate, and practice some stress-reducing activities.

There are lots of books on this subject on the market, thanks once more for selecting this one! Every effort was created to make sure it's stuffed with the maximum amount of helpful data as attainable, please enjoy!

The Alkaline Diet

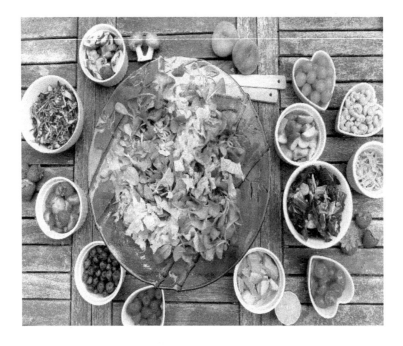

The main principle behind the diet is a philosophy that believes the foods we eat can easily alter the chemistry of our bodies. It all depends on if the food is alkaline or acidic. Basically, our body's pH will change depending on what foods we eat.

You need to understand that when our bodies need energy, it begins to burn food. This process is very controlled and takes place in an environment that our bodies control. When our bodies break down the foods we consume and get the energy from them, we are burning the foods but in a very controlled, slow way. This is what is known as your metabolism, the conversion of food into energy. This works a lot like a fire because it involves a chemical reaction to break down the food. These chemical reactions happen in a controlled and slow manner.

It is just like when you burn wood in your furnace when we burn foods, they are going to produce waste that is sometimes called "ash". This waste product could be either alkaline or acid.

These "ashes" are what alters the pH in our body. It all depends on the mineral, sulfur, or protein content in the food. Consuming foods that leave behind acidic ash like refined carbs, processed foods, fried foods, or sugar can, with time, increase inflammation and this leaves us vulnerable to disease. The bottom line is that if our bodies get exposed to huge amounts of acidic "ash", it will slowly begin to get more vulnerable to diseases because the immune system is getting weaker.

Our bodies house many organs that are very good at eliminating and neutralizing acid. There is a limit to the amount of acid our bodies can handle effectively. The Alkaline Diet doesn't try to change the pH in the blood but removes the stress of trying to maintain a healthy pH in the body by giving it the tools to thrive. Foods that form alkaline like plant proteins, tubers, vegetables, and whole fruits are all alkaline since they are anti-inflammatory, natural, fresh foods that are delicious and rich in antioxidants, chlorophyll, minerals, and vitamins. On the other hand, when our bloodstream gets impacted by a large level of alkalinity, it forms a protective layer that will try to keep our bodies healthy.

This diet is more of an eating plan rather than a diet. It is used to improve our health. Since it has an emphasis on fresh fruits and vegetables, its basis is on the idea that after the foods we eat get absorbed and digested, they will reach the kidneys as eight base- or acid-forming compounds.

There have been many techniques used to look at foods and figure out their base or acid load on the body. Some foods are going to be more base- or acid-producing than others. Surprisingly cheddar is more acid forming than egg whites. Spinach is more base-forming that watermelon.

It is thought that a diet that is high in foods that are acidic will disrupt the blood's pH level and then will trigger the loss of minerals like calcium while the body tries to restore its natural equilibrium. This imbalance is what causes us to be susceptible to illnesses.

The alkaline diet doesn't just help improve your health, it can slow the aging process, preserve muscle mass, and protect against many other health problems such as osteoporosis, kidney stones, cardiovascular disease, diabetes, and the common cold. This diet can also help you lose weight and boost your energy levels.

For these reasons, it is recommended that we try to choose foods that are high in alkalinity.

The following categorizes the various types of foods based on their "ashes".

- Alkaline: Foods like fruits, nuts, legumes, and vegetables.

- Neutral: Foods that contain starches, fats, and sugars

- Acidic: Foods like alcohol, eggs, grains, dairy, poultry, fish, and meats

Here is a bit of background about the alkalinity/acid of a normal diet and points about how this diet can help the human body:

- Researchers think that there has been a huge change from the hunger/gatherer civilization to what we have today. With the agricultural revolution and the mass industrialization of the foods we eat in the past 200 years, the foods we eat have a lot less chloride, magnesium, and potassium. It does have a lot more sodium as compared to other diets.

- Our kidneys keep the electrolyte levels normal. When the kidneys get exposed to very acidic substances, the electrolytes have to be used to fight acidity.

- The ratio of sodium and potassium in normal diets today has changed drastically. Potassium should outnumber sodium by ten to one but the ration has dwindled down to one to three. When eating a "normal" American diet, we now eat three times more sodium than potassium in an average day.

- These changes to our diets have caused an increase in metabolic acidosis. Basically this means the pH levels in our bodies aren't optimal anymore. Besides that, most people suffer from problems like magnesium and potassium deficiency.

- This causes the aging process to accelerate, degenerates bone and tissue mass, and the gradual loss in the functioning of organs. Because of the high degree of acid in our bodies it forces our bodies to get the minerals it needs from our tissues, organs, cells, and bones.

What is pH?

Let's begin with a little refresher in chemistry class and remind ourselves about what pH is. A simple definition is how much hydrogen ion concentration there is in our body. The initials pH is short of "power of hydrogen". The "p" stands for "potent" or the German word for power and "H" stands for the element symbol for hydrogen. The pH scale ranges from one to 14. Seven is neutral. A pH of less than seven will be acidic. Solutions that have a pH of more than seven are alkaline. In order for us to have good health, our bodies need to be a little bit alkaline. Our blood's pH and other cellular fluids should be around a pH of 7.365 to 7.45. It is important to realize that pH levels will vary a lot throughout the body. Some parts will be acidic while others will be alkaline. Basically, there isn't a set level. Our stomachs are loaded with hydrochloric acid and this gives it a pH of between 2 to 3.5. This makes it very acidic. It needs to be this acidic so it can break down the foods that we consume and kills harmful bacteria. Our saliva ranges from pH levels of 6.8 to 7.3. The skin has a pH level of 4 to 6.5. This acts as a protective barrier from the environment. Our urine has a pH that will vary from alkaline to acid. It all depends on what your body needs in order to balance our internal environment due to the foods we eat.

The measurement that is most important will be your blood's pH. It needs to keep in a very narrow range between 7.365 to 7.45. This might seem simple but instead of our pH operating within a mathematical scale, it operates within a logarithmic scale in multiples of ten. This means that it will take ten times the amount of alkalinity to be able to neutralize an acid. If there is a jump from six to seven, it might not seem like much but it will take ten times the amount of alkalinity to neutralize this amount. Basically, a pH of five will be 100 times more acidic than a pH of seven. A pH of four will be 1,000 times more acidic. Does this help you understand?

Don't begin stressing about staying in or falling out of that range. Remember our bodies are pretty great at regulating the pH of your blood. Our bodies don't "find" the balance. It has many parts that do this and keeps the blood's pH between 7.365 and 7.45 at all times. If you make poor lifestyle and diet choices, your body works harder to keep the balance. If you want to address the inflammation and acidity in your body by changing your dietary choices to foods that are more alkaline, it will help balance your system and bring your body back to its best vitality.

Even the smallest of alterations to the pH level of different organisms can cause massive problems. Because of the environmental concerns like increasing the deposition of CO_2 in the ocean, its pH level has dropped from 8.2 to 8.1 and the many different life forms that live in the ocean have suffered a lot. The pH level is critical for plant growth and it can affect the mineral content of foods we consume. The human body, soil, and minerals in the ocean are buffers that help maintain the optimal pH level. When there is a rise in acidity, minerals will fall.

- Blood pH

You know that the body is constantly working to make sure that you maintain healthy pH levels in your body. The tricky thing is, there are three liquids in the body that are typically at slightly different pH levels. Overall, they are mostly controlled by the same things. The first thing we are going to look at is blood pH.

Are normal pH range for your blood is 7.35 to 7.45. This means that the blood is normally naturally alkaline or basic. When compared to stomach acid, which is around 3 to 5.5, you can see the big difference. The stomach is supposed to be at this acidic level to break down the foods that you eat. Ironically, if stomach acid becomes more acidic or more basic, it can create the same symptoms of acid reflux, but that's a different discussion. This low pH helps you to digest food and destroys the germs that may enter your stomach.

What can cause the pH of your blood to change or hit levels that are abnormal?

Health problems are typically the most common cause of the blood become too alkaline or acidic. Also, a change in normal blood pH levels can signal a medical emergency or health condition. This can include:

- Poisoning

- Drug overdose

- Hemorrhage

- Shock

- Infection

- Gout

- Lung disease

- Kidney disease

- Heart disease

- Diabetes

- Asthma

Acidosis refers to when your blood pH level drops to anything below 7.35 and starts to become too acidic. Alkalosis refers to when your blood pH level increases to more than 7.45 and starts to become too alkaline. There are two main organs that work hard to help keep your blood pH levels normal:

- Kidneys – These organs work by remove the acid through your urine so that you excrete it.

- Lungs – These organs work by getting rid of carbon dioxide through your breathing.

The different forms of blood alkalosis and acidosis depend greatly on the reason for it. The top two causes are:

- Metabolic – These types of problems most often occur when your blood pH changes due to an issue of condition within the kidneys.

- Respiratory – These types of problems most often occur when your blood pH changes due to a breathing or lung condition.

It is normal for the blood pH levels to be tested as part of a blood gas test. This type of test is also sometimes referred to as an ABG test, or arterial blood gas test. It works by measuring how much carbon dioxide and oxygen is in your blood. Your general practitioner may choose to test your blood pH as a normal part of your year health screenings, or if you already suffer from certain health conditions. Blood pH tests do require having blood removed using a needle. The lab will be sent the blood sample, and perform the test.

There are at-home blood pH tests when you can do by pricking your finger. These tests won't provide you as accurate of a reading as a test at your doctor's office will. Using a urine pH litmus paper test will not provide you with your blood's pH level, but it can let you know if there is something that isn't right.

Let's take a moment to look more closely at some reasons why your blood pH levels my move out of the normal range.

High blood pH, also known as alkalosis, will happen if the pH of your blood rises above the normal range. There are many different causes for the high blood pH levels. You may have a temporary increase in your blood pH with simple illnesses. There are some foods that can also cause your blood to become more alkaline. There are also more serious causes to this alkalosis that can create further problems.

First off is fluid loss. Losing too much water can cause your blood pH levels to increase. This is due to the fact that you also lose some blood electrolytes, which are minerals and salts, when you lose water. These include potassium and sodium. Diarrhea, vomiting, and sweating can cause excess fluid loss. Medications and diuretic drugs can also cause a person to urinate more often, leading to higher blood pH levels. Treatment for fluid loss requires you to make sure you are getting plenty of fluids and making sure you electrolytes are replaced. Some sport drinks can you accomplish this. Your doctor may also look at your medications and stop any that may be causing the fluid loss.

Next, kidney problems can cause high blood pH levels. Your kidneys play a large role in keeping your blood pH normal. A kidney problem can then cause an accumulation of alkalinity in your blood. This is due to the fact that the kidneys won't remove any excess alkaline substances through your urine. For example, the kidneys could improperly filter bicarbonate back into the blood. There are medications and other treatments that can help to lower your blood pH levels.

When there is blood acidosis, it can affect the way every organ in your body functions. Low blood pH is more common issue than high blood pH. Acidosis is often a warning sign to some health problem that is not being controlled.

There are some health conditions that can cause natural acids to build up within the blood. Some forms of acids that can end of lowering blood pH include:

- Carbonic acid

- Hydrochloric acid

- Phosphoric acid

- Sulphuric acid

- Keto acids

- Lactic acid

An improper diet can cause problems. Eating a diet that is imbalanced can create a temporary low blood pH level. Not eating enough or going for extended periods of time without eating can create more acid in the blood. Try to avoid eating too many acid-forming foods, which include:

- Grains – rice, pasta, bread, and flour

- Fish

- Meat

- Eggs

- Poultry – turkey and chicken

- Dairy – yogurt, cheese, and cow's milk

You balance your blood pH by eating more alkaline-forming foods. These most often include dried, frozen, and fresh fruit, and fresh and cooked veggies. Stay far away from fad diets or starvation diets. When trying to lose weight, do so in a healthy, safe way following a balanced diet.

Another cause for low pH levels in the blood is due to diabetic ketoacidosis. If you suffer from diabetes, you blood can end up becoming acidic if you don't properly regular your blood sugar levels. Diabetic ketoacidosis occurs when the body is unable to make enough insulin or use it properly.

Insulin helps by moving sugar from the foods that we eat into the cells of the body. This is where the body will then burn it as fuel. If insulin is unable to be used, you body starts to break down the stored fat in your body to power itself. This releases an acid wasted known as ketones. If the body is not able to regulate this process, the acid will build up and trigger low blood pH.

It is important that you seek out emergency care if your blood sugar level is over 300 milligrams per deciliter. If you suffer from any of the following symptoms, speak with your doctor:

- Confusion

- Stomach pain

- Fruity-smelling breath

- Shortness of breath

- Vomiting or nausea

- Weakness or fatigue

- Frequent urination

- Excess thirst

Diabetic ketoacidosis is most often a sign that diabetes is not being treated properly and is out of control. This can sometimes be the first signs of diabetes for some. Making sure your diabetes is well treated will help keep your blood pH balanced. It may require a strict diet and exercise plan, insulin injections, and medications in order to stay healthy.

A third cause of low blood pH is metabolic acidosis. This is when low blood pH is caused by kidney disease or failure. This occurs when the kidneys are unable to remove acids from your body through urination. This will increase the acids in your body and lower your blood pH.

The most common symptoms of metabolic acidosis are:

- Heavy breathing

- Fast heartbeat

- Headache pain

- Vomiting and nausea

- Loss of appetite

- Weakness and fatigue

Treatment for this problem will often include medications to help the kidneys work better. In more serious cases, it may require a kidney transplant or dialysis. Dialysis works by cleaning the blood.

The last cause of low blood pH is respiratory acidosis. When the lungs aren't functioning probably to remove carbon dioxide quickly from the body, the blood pH levels will lower. This will most often happen if a person suffers from a chronic or serious lung condition, such as:

- Diaphragm disorders

- Chronic obstructive pulmonary disease

- Pneumonia

- Bronchitis

- Sleep apnea

- Asthma

People who are obese, have had surgery, or who abuse opioid painkillers or sedatives are at a higher risk of developing respiratory acidosis. In some cases, the kidneys are able to pick up the slack and remove the excess blood acids through excretion. A person may need to be given extra oxygen and medications like steroids and bronchodilators to help the lungs function properly. In really serious cases, mechanical ventilation and intubation may have to be used in those with respiratory acidosis in order to bring the blood pH back to normal.

- Urine pH

The next type of pH we are going to look at is urine pH. Urine is made up of waste products, salts, and water that are excreted through the kidneys. The balance of these different compounds can affect the acidity level of the urine.

According to the American Association for Clinical Chemistry, the average pH of urine is 6.0, but it can range from 4.5 to 8.0. Any levels under 5.0 is considered acidic urine, and any levels above 8.0 is considered basic urine.

Sometimes different laboratories will have different ranges as to what they consider to be normal pH levels for the urine.

One of the main things that affects the pH of your urine is the things that you eat. If you go to the doctor, they will often ask what foods you have eaten before they evaluate the results of a urine pH test.

If, before a test, you have eaten more acid-form foods, you urine is going to be more acidic. The same goes for having eaten more alkaline foods. If a person has extremely high pH levels in their urine, which means it is more alkaline, it could be a sign of some medical conditions, like:

- Urinary tract infections

- Kidney stones

- Other kidney-related disorders

A person can also have high urine pH levels if they have experienced prolonged vomiting. Vomiting causes the body to get rid of stomach acid, which causes of the bodily fluids to become more basic.

When urine is acidic, it creates an environment conducive for kidney stones, as well. When the urine is acidic, it can also be a sign of several severe medical conditions, like:

- Starvation

- Diarrhea

- Diabetic ketoacidosis

As you will notice, much of this is the same of the pH levels of the blood. There are also certain medications that can affect the pH of the urine. Sometimes doctors will have a patient withhold certain medications the day or night before they are going to have a urinalysis.

- Saliva pH

The last pH we are going to look at is saliva pH. The normal pH range for saliva is 6.2 to 7.6. The things you drink and eat can change the pH of your saliva. For example, the bacteria in the mouth breaks down the carbohydrates that you eat, which releases aspartic acid, butyric acid, and lactic acid. This will lower your saliva pH levels. Age also plays a big role in this. Adults will often have more acidic saliva pH levels than children do.

Just like every other area of your body, your mouth needs to keep a balanced pH. Your saliva pH levels can drop to lower than 5.5 when you have been drinking a lot of acidic beverages. When this occurs, the acids in your mouth will begin to break down your tooth enamel.

If your tooth enamel becomes too thin, your dentin will then be exposed. This can end up causing discomfort when you consume sugar, cold, or hot beverages. Just to give you an example of foods and drinks that can do this, here are some numbers:

- Cherries have a pH of 4

- American cheese has a pH of 5

- White wine has a pH of 4

- Soft drinks have a pH of 3

It's easy to spot unbalanced saliva pH levels. Some of the most common indicators are:

- Tooth cavities

- Sensitivity to cold or hot beverages or food

- Persistent bad breath

If you want, you can even test the pH of your saliva. In order to test the pH of your saliva, you will need to find some pH strips. These can easily be found online or in drugstores. Once you have your strips, this is what you do:

- Make sure you don't eat or drink anything for at least two hours before testing.

- Allow your mouth to fill with saliva and then swallow this or spit it out.

- Allow your mouth to fill with saliva again and then place a small amount on one of your pH strips.

- The strip will then react to your saliva. It will change colors based on how alkaline or acidic your saliva is. The container that your pH strips came should show you a color chart. Place your strip next to the chart to match up the colors and find out what your saliva's pH level is.

In order to make sure that you saliva pH stays balanced it's important that you eat foods that are in a healthy pH range. It's also important that you don't let yourself be deprived of important vitamins and minerals. There are some more efficient ways to make sure that your saliva pH remains balanced.

- Stay away from sugary soft drinks. If you must drink them, try to drink them quickly and chase them with some water. Sipping sugary drinks over a long period of time does more damage.

- Limit your black coffee. Adding in some creamy, non-sugary, can help to cut the acidity of the coffee.

- Avoid brushing your teeth immediately after consuming high-acidic drinks like beer, wine, cider, fruit juices, or soft drinks. These types of drinks will soften up your tooth enamel. If you brush too soon after consuming these things, you will further damage your enamel.

- Chew some sugar less gum after you have consumed any beverages or food. Chewing gum will cause your mouth to produce more saliva and it will help to bring your pH level back to normal. It is also believed that xylitol can prevent bacteria from sticking to your tooth enamel.

- Keep yourself hydrated so make sure you drink plenty of water.

Harmful Effects of an Imbalanced pH

You should know how important it is to maintain a balanced pH. This section will tell you about the fatal consequences of changes to the pH. If the pH level in the body gets too alkaline, a symptom called Alkalosis is going to happen. When the body is put under these conditions, you will begin to experience a loss of electrolytes, liver disease, lower oxygen levels, etc. Here are some symptoms of alkalosis:

- Tingling in the face

- Problems breathing

- Seizure

- Sudden onset of muscle spasms

- Twitching

- Light-headedness

- Confusion

On the other hand, if the body starts to get too acidic, your body will enter into a state of acidosis. There are some risks to acidosis like:

- Lethargy

- Breathlessness

- Fatigue

- Confusion

- Kidney damage

- Insulin resistance

- Diabetes

- Increased risk of heart disease

- Renal complications

- Lactic imbalance

- Respiratory problems

- Metabolic problems

Acidosis can be brought on by a diet that isn't balanced and that contains a lot of animal products with only a few vegetables and fruits. Here are some symptoms of acidosis:

- Vomiting

- Nausea

- Increased heart rate

- Arrhythmia

- Diarrhea

- Muscle weakness

- Seizures

- Coughing

- Shortness of breath

- Confusion

- Sleepiness

- Headache

- Loss of consciousness

- Coma

The Alkaline Lifestyle

Studies have been shown that when acidosis is induced and caused by the diet, it is an actual phenomenon. It needs to be recognized and treated, it can be treated by changes to the diet and has significant relevance.

Here are some conditions that the Alkaline Diet could help prevent:

- Heart disease, stroke, and hypertension

A diet high in acidic foods has been associated with higher mortality rates. Researchers studied over 44,000 men and 36,000 women in a 15 year time span. With both women and men, they showed higher mortality rates in the ones who ate a high acid-based diet as compared to ones who ate a diet rich in fresh vegetable and fruits.

Another study in 2016 found that people who had high PRAL had an increase in developing atherosclerotic cardiovascular disease and were put into a high risk group as compared to people who had lower PRAL scores.

Around 33% of adults are diagnosed with high blood pressure. This condition will increase the danger for stroke and cardiovascular disease. There are several risk factors for cardiopathy and high blood pressure, as well as being overweight and inactive. There are very distinct and clear links between the risks and the foods you eat. A normal American diet is known to be high in animal products and very low in vegetables and fruits. It can cause low urine pH and metabolic acidosis. High dietary acid could cause hypertension and could increase the risk of heart disease. Basically, the alkaline diet is high in magnesium and potassium that promotes healthy blood pressure. Consuming more alkalizing foods could shift the number of minerals in your body and could decrease the risk of heart disease.

- Kidney stones

One in ten people will have problems with kidney stones in their lifetime. There are several risk factors involved but a diet that is high in sugar, sodium, and protein could increase the risk by adding more nutrients that promote stones than the kidneys will be able to filter. This is very true in diets that are high in sodium that will increase how much calcium your kidneys have to filter. Foods that promote stones include uric acid that is found in animal proteins, phosphorus, sodium, oxalate that is found in chocolate and some nuts, and calcium. These can all contribute to a low-grade metabolic acidosis. Healthy, young people can filter these foods, when we begin aging, we will experience a decline in kidney function. Passing kidney stones isn't a picnic and new research shows that dietary acid load is a great way to predict stone formation. Basically, when you add more nutrient rich and alkalizing foods, you could reduce the stone promoters from getting bigger.

Eating a diet heavy in acidic foods can increase metabolic acidosis and this in turn can increase the risk of kidney disease. One study followed over 15,000 people who didn't have kidney disease for 21 years. These people were already at a high risk for developing atherosclerosis. After they adjusted for factors such as demographics and caloric intake, they found that participants who consumed foods that were more acidic had a higher risk of developing chronic kidney disease.

Some of the dietary components like getting protein from vegetable sources and a higher intake of magnesium protected against chronic kidney disease.

- Chronic low back pain

Research is still being done on this but there is a bit of evidence that indicates that chronic back pain could improve by adding in a supplement of alkalizing minerals. Increasing magnesium by taking supplements helps the enzyme system function better and activates vitamin D. This will, in turn, improve your back pain. Basically, if you have back pain, following the alkaline diet will give your level of magnesium a boost and might ease your symptoms.

- Type 2 diabetes

Around tenth of the adult population within the U.S. has been diagnosed with a kind of a pair of polygenic disease (Type 2 diabetes). This is an upset that may cause your glucose to rise. This can cause your cells to become resistant to insulin. Type two polygenic disorder is preventable and analysis has shown that dietary acid load has been related to multiplied risk. Basically, it has also been shown that in addition to helping you keep a healthy weight, a diet that promotes alkaline foods might cut back the danger of developing type 2 of the polygenic disorder.

During a study in Germany in 2014, researchers followed 66,485 women for 14 years prior. Within that time there was 1,372 new cases of diabetes that was diagnosed. The researchers analyzed their food intake and determined that the women who ate diet that were high in acid based foods had higher risks of developing diabetes. The researchers suggest that high intake of foods that are acidic might be linked to insulin resistance which has been linked to diabetes.

- Osteoporosis

Osteoporosis is a progressive bone disease that is characterized by a lower than normal bone mineral content. This is a common problem for postmenopausal women and will dramatically increase a person's risk of fractures. It is believed that in order to keep your blood pH constant, the body will start to take alkaline minerals, like calcium, out of the bones to buffer the excess acids when excessive acid-forming foods are consumed.

According to this believe, acid-forming diets, like that standard Western diet, will end up causing a los in bone density. This is what they refer to as "acid-ash hypothesis of osteoporosis." However, there is one problem with this theory, it leaves out the function of the kidneys, which play an important part in removing acids from the body and regulates body pH. The kidneys make what is known as bicarbonate ions that help to neutralize acids that are in your blood to help the body closely mange the pH of the blood.

The respiratory system also kicks into action when there are excess acid levels. When the bicarbonate ions that your kidneys produce binds to the acids within your blood, they create what is known as carbon dioxide, which is then breathed that out, and water, which is excreted. This theory also ignores that the main cause of osteoporosis is a loss in the protein collagen within the bones. Ironically, having a loss in collagen has often been linked to low levels of ascorbic acid and orthosilicic acid.

It's important that you keep in mind that scientific evident that links dietary acid to bone density or fracture risk is a mixed bag. While there have been many observational studies that haven't found any association, others have found many significant links. Clinical trials, which are often the most accurate, have found that acid-forming diets don't have a large impact on calcium levels within the body.

While scientific studies may be mixed, there are still plenty of people who say the standard Western diet does impose a high acid load, which can affect bone health. To lower this risk of osteoporosis, it is important that people consume seven to nine servings of vegetables and fruits each day to help keep the pH balanced so that the body never feels it necessary to take calcium from the bones.

- Muscle mass

When we age, we will lose muscle mass, and it will be more prominent if you lead an inactive lifestyle. Having less muscle mass will mean you burn fewer calories throughout the day and this contributes to that "weight creep" that many people will develop as they age. Losing muscle mass will make you more susceptible to fracturing a bone if we fall and this could hinder your independence. A diet rich in alkaline vegetables and fruits can reduce the net acid load in older adults this can result in preserving muscle mass. Basically, everybody wants their independence when aging and adding in a serving of vegetables and fruits to every meal could help.

During a three year research that involved 384 women and men that were aged 65 and older showed that eating a lot of foods that are rich in potassium like fresh vegetables and fruits might help adults maintain their muscle mass as they age. In recent studies, researchers looked at data collected in 2013 from a group of 2,689 women who were aged from 18 to 79 and found a significant association between following the alkaline diet and keeping muscle mass. A diet rich in alkaline vegetables and fruits can reduce the net acid load in older adults this can result in preserving muscle mass. Basically, everybody wants their independence when aging and adding in a serving of vegetables and fruits to every meal could help.

- Chemotherapy and cancer

Even though acidosis caused by diet could increase the risk for cancer, right now there isn't any research that the alkaline could prevent cancer. Some studies have shown that when you eat more foods that promote alkalinity, the pH in the urine could be changed to help how effective chemotherapy drugs work. If you been diagnosed with cancer and are taking chemotherapy, talk with your doctor or dietitian before changing your diet. Basically, it would be best if you eat a diet that has an emphasis on plant foods, consuming between five and nine servings of vegetables and fruits every day, and don't consume a lot of red meat, processed meats, alcohol, and sodium which is a lot like the alkaline diet.

A normal American diet leaves a lot to be desired and this leaves our bodies short of many essential minerals and vitamins. If this is left unchecked, for a short amount of time, it could make you feel tired, cause weight gain, change your concentration levels and mood, and disrupt sleep. For longer amounts of your time, imbalances within the diet may cause chronic diseases like kidney stones, heart condition, type two polygenic disease, and high-pressure level. Giving your body a mixture of nutrient-dense foods daily will give it a chance to fight against the disease.

If you have been diagnosed with any health conditions like cancer or kidney disease, make sure you talk with your health care provider before changing your diet. If you take medicines that change how the body absorbs potassium, calcium, or other minerals you need to check with your doctor before starting this diet.

Following the food list too strictly without taking into consideration factors such as overall calorie intake or protein could cause other health problems such as excessive weight loss or nutrient deficiency.

An alkaline diet should never be used instead of normal treatment for any health problem, adopting a diet that is rich in vegetables and fruits might help protect you against specific diseases and have better health overall.

There are many foods on the foods list such as nuts, beans, and grains that have great attributes and then the foods such as wine and coffee need to be consumed in moderation. Instead of looking at the foods as ones to eat and what to avoid, think about the base and acid forming foods and try to have a balanced diet.

80/20 Rule

When you decide to get healthy, you can't expect to be perfect on the first day and you can't deprive yourself of foods that you really enjoy. To have success when learning to eat alkaline and keeping this lifestyle, you need to learn moderation since life is about balance. Deprivation is the reason behind the failures of most diets. Finding the perfect balance can be confusing and challenging when you first begin this new lifestyle. In order to get the most benefits out of the alkaline diet is to use the 80/20 rule. This means that in order to keep a healthy internal environment, you need to try to eat a diet that contains around 80 percent alkaline-forming foods and the remaining 20 percent coming from acid-forming foods. Basically, refined starches and animal proteins are acid, whereas, fruits, vegetables, and beans are alkaline.

It is easy to put this into play if you just visualize your plate and think about food groups. To have optimal health, you need to eat plant proteins, healthy fats, tubers, vegetables, and fruits that take up 80 percent of your plate. Other acidic foods and starches will take the remaining 20 percent. If you can do this for every meal, this will guarantee your diet will always be 80 percent alkaline and 20 percent acid. You might be tempted to get rid of all alkaline foods from your diet. This would be a huge mistake. High protein foods like beans, fish, milk, and meat are acidifying but your body has to have protein so it can repair and rebuild your body.

If you like tofu that is mildly alkaline and low acid then go ahead and put it into your diet. Just eat it in moderation. Even though it isn't a high protein food, you can even have a piece of chocolate or a slice of birthday cake every now and then. The key words are moderation, balance, and shifting your diet from constantly eating acid-forming foods to a diet where they begin taking up a small part of your plate. Slowly bring back in foods that have the most impact and before you realize what is happening, all that good will outweigh the bad and your energy and health will increase.

Exercise

Another essential component to help manage stress, keeping a healthy weight, and decreasing the risk of chronic disease is physical activity. Here is a guideline for persons over six years old:

- Adolescents and Children

    - Adolescents and children need to include bone and muscle-strengthening activities for one hour each day for three days per week.

    - One hour a day needs to be either vigorous or moderate-intensity aerobic activity. There should be a vigorous activity done three days per week.

    - Adolescents and children need to perform one hour or more of physical activity each day.

- Adults

    - For substantial advantages, adults have to do about seventy-five minutes per week of vigorous intensity or no less than a hundred and fifty minutes per week of moderate-intensity exercise or an equal combination of these two. Aerobic exercises need to be performed in a series of ten minutes intervals.

- For in-depth benefits, adults have to increase their aerobic activity to three hundred minutes per week or one hundred fifty minutes of vigorous intensity activity per week.

- Adults have to do muscle-strengthening activities that involve each major muscle cluster for 2 days or a lot weekly.

• Older Adults

- If an older adult can't do a hundred and fifty minutes per week of moderate-intensity activity because of chronic conditions, they need to be physically active if their conditions and ability allow it.

While we all know that we need to exercise, we may not completely understand why we should and what it can do for us. Let's take a look at some of the many benefits regular exercise can provide:

1. It can increase your energy levels – Exercise is able to improve both the efficiency and strength of your cardiovascular system to help send nutrients and oxygen to your muscles. When the cardiovascular systems works more efficiently, everything else seems easier and you will find that you have more energy for the things you enjoy doing.

2. It can improve your muscle strength – When you stay active, it keeps your muscles strong and your ligaments, joints, and tendons flexible. This allows you to move more easily and keeps you from injuring yourself. When you have strong ligaments and muscles, you help to reduce your risk of lower back and joint pain by keeping everything in proper alignment. This will also end up improving your balance and coordination.

3. It helps you to keep a healthy weight – Exercise helps you to burn calories. In addition, the more muscle mass you have, you will increase your metabolic rate. This means that you burn more calories at rest. This will help to boost your self-esteem and help you to lose weight.

4. It improves the function of the brain – Exercise improves your oxygen levels and blood flow to the brain. It will also encourage the release of hormones that help with the production of cells within the hippocampus, which is the area of the brain that helps with learning and memory. This will then help to boost your cognitive ability and concentration level, and it lowers you risk of cognitive degenerative diseases like Alzheimer's

5. It helps your heart – Exercise helps to your reduce your LDL levels, which is what clogs your arteries. It increases your HDL levels and lowers your blood pressure, so the stress on your heart is reduced. It also helps to strengthen the muscles of your heart. When you combine this with a healthy diet, exercise is able to lower your risk of coronary heart disease.

6. It lowers your risk for type 2 diabetes – Exercising regularly helps keep your blood glucose levels under control, which delays or prevents the onset of diabetes. Exercise will also help to prevent obesity, which is the main factor in diabetes.

7. Improves the immune system – Exercise helps the body to pump oxygen and nutrients through the body that it needs to help fuel the cells that fight off viruses and bacteria.

8. It helps to reduce the chance of developing degenerative bone disease – Exercises that are weight bearing, like weight training, walking, or running, helps to lower your risk of osteoporosis and osteoarthritis.

9. It can help to reduce some cancers – Being fit could mean that it could reduce your risk of breast cancer, colon cancer, and maybe even lung and endometrial cancers. According to studies performed by Seattle Cancer Research Center, they suggest that 35% of all cancer related deaths were linked to being sedentary and overweight.

10. It helps you sleep better – Being physically active makes you tired, thus, you will be ready for bed. Having good sleep quality helps to improve your overall wellness and it can help to reduce stress.

11. You will have a better mood and wellbeing – Exercise is able to help stimulate the release of endorphins which will make you feel even better and feel relaxed. These endorphins will also work to improve your mood and lower stress.

12. It can help treat or prevent mental illness – Exercise has the power to help your meet others, lower stress, provides you a sense of achievement, cope with frustration, and provide you with that all important "me time," all of this can help you prevent depression.

Advantages

Here is a rundown of all the advantages the alkaline diet offers your body:

- It can increase your sex drive and enhances sexual power.

- It can slow down the natural aging process and will keep you looking fresher and younger.

- It can improve the health of your teeth and gums.

- The alkaline diet can increase your body's available energy and will keep it energized throughout the day.

- It will help you lose weight.

- It can help improve your body's immunity and can protect you from developing cancer.

- It can help boost how the body absorbs vitamins and minimizes the deficiency of magnesium.

- It can help lower chronic pain and inflammation.

- It will lower the risk of stroke and hypertension.

- It can help protect bone mass and muscle density.

Foods and Your Body

Scientists have known for some time now that what makes up our diets can affect the acid balance in our bodies. Changes in the acidity of your urine that are brought on by changes in your diet have always been interesting to physiologists. This shows the role kidneys play in maintaining homeostasis or the state of balance within our bodies. Research from the Paleolithic era shows the drastic changes in the diet as compared to ones of our ancestors who were hunter-gatherers and the rise of chronic diseases.

Michael Pollan's guideline of "Eat food, not too much, mostly plants" is quoted often but isn't followed that often. Most of 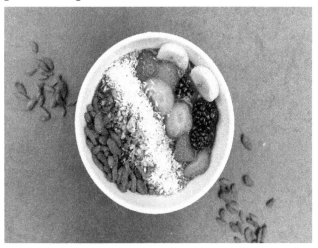 the Americans' calories come from processed foods that don't have any valuable nutrients but are extremely high in unhealthy fats, added sugars, and sodium. These foods are coupled with large amounts of animal proteins and very low intake of vegetables and fruits. It isn't a surprise that this diet causes diseases but we don't know why. One reason is the modern diet exchanged magnesium and potassium-rich foods for salt. This creates a deficiency of potassium within the diet and this increases the acid load inside the body.

What's worse is with time, a diet high in acid will produce a "low grade chronic metabolic acidosis". This means we are constantly in a state of inflammation and high acidity. Since our bodies have to operate in a stable pH, it has to neutralize a very high dietary acid load that puts a strain on our body's buffering system. The consequences for our body constantly attempting to keep a constant pH within the high acidic environment will lead to wasting muscle and increased chronic diseases.

Acute inflammation like our bodies responding to a cut or fever is necessary for health. Chronic inflammation, on the other hand, is a normal process that has gone very wrong. It has a domino effect that could seriously undermine our health. Good news is, what you put in your mouth will affect your inflammation levels. Eating foods like spices and herbs will help reduce the inflammation in the body and this is the best way to protect your health.

When you can lower the acid-producing foods in your diet and replace it with alkaline-producing foods, this can lower acid levels and will reduce the strain on our body's natural buffering system. Reducing the acid load in the body might delay or prevent kidney stones from forming, improve heart health by promoting a healthier blood pressure, lowering your risk for type 2 diabetes, and maintaining muscle mass. Employing some strategies to help neutralize your diet might mean a difference between a healthy, disease-free body and chronic low-grade acidosis.

Alkaline Water

You might have heard about alkaline water. This type of water is less acidic than even tap water and it is a lot better. Alkaline water is rich in bicarbonate, magnesium, potassium, silica, and calcium. Normal tap water is normally neutral. It has a pH of about seven. Alkaline water will have a pH of about eight or nine. Alkaline water can be found at most grocery stores, and you can find water ionizer in many large chain stores, too. Regular water is great for the majority of people since there isn't scientific evidence that verifies all the claims that alkaline water brags about. The current research claiming alkaline water can help treat chronic acidosis, reduces liver damage, improves gut health, protects from toxins, improves health overall, is not convincing. It is also believed to help slow down the ageing process and keep your pH levels regulated.

To get alkaline water, regular water has to go through ionization process. This process increases the pH level of the water. There are many different ways you can increase the alkaline properties in your water by using additives, faucet attachments, and filters. These are things you can do at home which may be cheaper than buying bottled alkaline water. In a study published in the *Annals of Otology, Rhinology & Laryngology*, alkaline water that has a pH of 8.8 could actually help soothe acid reflux symptoms because the acid is due to high levels of pepsin, and the pH of alkaline water has the ability to kill the enzyme. Pepsin, by the way, is a natural enzyme that the body uses to break down food proteins. In another study published in the *Journal of the International Society of Sports Nutrition* has found a significant different in the blood viscosity in those who consumed high pH water as compared to regular water after a strenuous workout. In yet another study, this one published in the *Shanghai Journal of Preventive Medicine*, found that alkaline water could benefit those who suffer from diabetes, high cholesterol, and high blood pressure.

It's possible that drinking alkaline water could provide some benefits for some, but studies haven't produced evidence that it will benefit your health. People who have kidney disease or who take specific medications that change the function of the kidneys are cautioned against it since the minerals in alkaline water might add up in the body. If you don't have kidney problems, you might think about drinking alkaline water. Water that has naturally occurring minerals will be your best bet as a source for alkaline water.

While there may not be a large amount of proven scientific research concerning alkaline water, there is still many proponents who believe that alkaline water can provide you with the following:

1. Alkaline water has better hydrating properties than normal tap water. This makes it beneficial for people who work out regularly and need more water in their body. From a scientific viewpoint, the water molecules within alkaline

water are smaller and your cells are able to more easily absorb them, which helps to re-hydrate the body.

2. Alkaline water can also boost your immunity. Having a healthy immune system can help to neutralize the acidity in your body, which can be caused by environmental toxins, stress, and a poor diet.

3. Alkaline water also contains different minerals like calcium and magnesium, both of which are extremely important for keeping your bones healthy.

4. Alkaline water also contains potent antioxidants that help to stop the growth of cell damaging free radicals within the body, which can increase the ageing process.

5. One of the best benefits of drinking alkaline water is that it can help to neutralize the acidity in the body by lowering the excessive acid content in the gastrointestinal tract and the stomach.

If you want to start consuming alkaline water, you don't have to go to the store and buy packages of the expensive alkaline water. You can make your own right at home. You can use baking soda to make you own alkaline water. Baking soda has a pH of 9. Mix in a half of a tablespoon of baking soda to a gallon of water. Shake it to make sure that the baking soda dissolves. Once dissolves, enjoy a cup. Make sure you stick to these measurements. While baking soda is good for you, you can overdose on it.

You can also make alkaline water using lemon. While lemon is considered acidic with a pH below 7, when it is added to water, or consumed and metabolized, it has an alkalizing effect and raises the body's pH. This is why you should always kick start you day with a glass of lemon water. There is no right or wrong way with this one. Add as much lemon juice as you like to your water and enjoy.

Alkaline Foods

There are many foods that are easy to tell whether they belong in the alkaline or acid category but there are also foods that are so evident. Let's look at a lemon. A lemon has a very tart taste so it is obviously acidic. Wrong, the nature of lemon is acidic, when the body metabolizes it, it becomes alkalizing. Foods that have a natural acidity don't always remain acidic once they have been eaten. Acidic foods such as sauerkraut, kefir, and citrus are alkalizing and very healing. What makes it even more confusing, many charts that show alkalizing and acidifying foods just use the words "alkaline foods" and "acid foods". This doesn't give an accurate picture in any way.

In order to be able to accurately predict the base or acid potential of any food, scientists have worked a long time to come up with a technique that uses the food's nutrient composition and determines what the baseload or true acid that goes into our bodies.

This brought about the PRAL or potential renal acid load scale. A PRAL score that is negative shows food that is alkaline or basic. If the PRAL score is positive, it shows that the foods are acidic. If the score shows zero, the food will be neutral. If the score is negative, then the food is alkaline. If you add up the PRAL values for every food that you eat during the day, you will get your net alkaline or acid load. While it isn't necessary to micromanage your diet to find the lowest PRAL score, it might be interesting to figure out your PRAL values are on any given day.

To example this further, PRAL measures the acidity or alkalinity of a food based on the amount of phosphorus, minerals, and protein that is leaves behind within the body once your body has metabolized it. Since phosphorus and protein break down into phosphoric acid and sulfuric acid, they believe to be acidifying to the body. When you metabolize an alkaline food, it leaves behind trace amounts of alkaline minerals, like potassium, magnesium, and calcium.

Here is a list of foods and their PRAL score to give you an idea of what this all means:

- Fruits:

    o Watermelon : -1.9

    o Strawberries: -2.2

    o Raisins: -21

    o Pineapple: -2.7

- Pear: -2.9

- Peach: -2.4

- Orange: -2.7

- Mango: -3.3

- Lemon: -2.6

- Kiwi fruit: -4.1

- Grapes: -3.9

- Grapefruit: -3.5

- Dried figs: -18.1

- Cherries: -3.6

- Black currants: -6.5

- Bananas: -5.5

- Apricots: -4.8

- Apples: -2.2

- Fish & Seafood

  - Zander: 7.1

  - Trout: 10.8

  - Tiger prawn: 18.2

  - Sole: 7.4

- Shrimp: 7.6

- Sardines: 13.5

- Herring: 8

- Salmon: 9.4

- Rose-fish: 10

- Prawn: 15.3

- Mussels: 15.3

- Halibut: 7.8

- Eel: 11

- Cod: 7.1

- Carp: 7.9

- Nuts

  - Walnuts: 6.8

  - Sweet almonds: 4.3

  - Pistachio: 8.5

  - Peanuts: 8.3

  - Hazelnuts: -2.8

- Fats & Oil

  - Sunflower seed oil: 0

- Olive oil: 0

- Margarine: -0.5

- Butter: 0.6

- Beverages

  - Dry white wine: -1.2

  - Vegetable juice: -3.6

  - Tomato juice: -2.8

  - Tea: -0.3

  - Red wine: -2.4

  - Unsweetened orange juice: -2.9

  - Mineral water: -0.1

  - Lemon juice: -2.5

  - Herbal tea: -0.2

  - Green tea: -0.3

  - Unsweetened grape juice: -1

  - Fruit tea: -0.3

  - Espresso: -2.3

  - Coffee: -1.4

  - Cocoa with semi-skimmed milk: -0.4

- Coca-cola: 0.4

- Carrot juice: -4.8

- Beetroot juice: -3.9

- Beer, stout: -0.1

- Beer, pale: 0.9

- Beer, draft: -0.2

- Unsweetened apple juice: -2.2

- Grains

  - Wheat flour: 6.9

  - Rye flour: 5.9

  - Rice, white: 1.7

  - Rice, brown: 12.5

  - Millet: 8.6

  - Corn: 3.9

- Bread

  - White bread: 3.7

  - Pumpernickel: 4.2

- Dairy Products and Eggs

  - Whey: -1.6

- Kefir: 0

- Parmesan: 34.2

- Plain yogurt: 1.5

- Gouda: 18.6

- Egg: 8.2

- Meats

  - Lean beef: 7.8

  - Chicken: 8.7

  - Duck: 4.1

  - Goose: 13

  - Pork sausage: 7

  - Salami: 11.6

  - Turkey: 9.9

- Sweets

  - White sugar: 0

  - Brown sugar: -1.2

  - Milk chocolate: 2.4

  - Honey: -0.3

- Veggies

- o   Onions: -1.5

- o   Brussels sprouts: -4.5

- o   Garlic: -1.7

- o   Potatoes: -4

- o   Soy beans: -3.4

- o   Mushrooms: -1.4

- o   Lettuce: -2.5

- o   Kohlrabi: -5.5

- o   Zucchini: -4.6

- Herbs & Vinegar

  - o   Parsley: -12

  - o   Apple cider vinegar: -2.3

  - o   Basil: -7.3

  - o   Chives: -5.3

As you can see, the foods that rank most alkaline on this scale are the veggies and fruits, and one nut. The foods that are most acidic are poultry, eggs, grains, seafood, and dairy products.

I really hate to be the bearer of bad news, but parmesan cheese ranks at +34.2 on the PRAL scale. This means that it is one of the most acidifying foods in the standard diet. Now, you may be wondering how on Earth dairy could be acidic since it contains calcium, which is one of the alkaline minerals. The reason for the acidity in dairy is due to its phosphorus content. It contains more phosphorus than it does calcium, making it acidic.

A quick note to make sure there isn't any confusing, the PRAL table measures the acidity of food in a different way to than how the pH of your blood is measured.

If we were to look at the PRAL scores on a regular pH scale, the 7.8 score of beef would mean that it is alkaline or neutral instead of acidic. Unlike the pH scale that we talked about earlier, a food on the PRAL scale that has a negative score actually means that it has more alkaline producing properties.

Foods to Avoid

When you want to restore the balance of pH in your body, you have to know what foods to eat and the ones to stay away from. A food's tendency to form acid in our bodies doesn't have anything to do with the food's natural pH. Instead, foods get classified according to the minerals that they release into the urine. When you are beginning, use the list below to help you decide about which of these foods you want to include into your 20 percent or stay away from them totally.

- Sodium

It is recommended that Americans only consume 2,300 milligrams of sodium or less each day. Just about anyone could benefit from less sodium in their diet because of its negative impact on our hearts. Sodium can be sneaky. It shows up in the majority of the foods we consume each day even if you don't shake a saltshaker. Since it is acid-forming, try to find unprocessed fresh foods that will keep your sodium low.

- Alcohol

Just a small amount of alcohol will have an effect on your body. Once you drink, the alcohol gets absorbed into the bloodstream and goes all through the body where it stays until the liver has time to process it. Out of the four macronutrients, only three of them can be stored in the body. These are fat, carbohydrates, and protein. The fourth one, alcohol, can't. For this reason alone, it will take priority over everything to be metabolized. When the body does this, all the other processes that need to take place get interrupted. Alcohol doesn't have any nutrients and is looked at as toxic waste by the body and should only be consumed in moderation.

- Grains

The grains that are consumed the most in the United States are wheat and corn. Both of these are very acidic. Once they are consumed and the body metabolizes them, they will produce acids that the liver has to get rid of. Wheat contains gluten which is a protein that many people with celiac disease or gluten intolerance can't digest. Since this protein can't get broken down, the body will attack it like an allergen and this can cause cramping, bloating, and gas. All grains are not equal. Some are alkaline like wild rice, quinoa, millet, and amaranth. Most of the grains that Americans eat are in products made with corn or refined flour. Refined grains don't have any fiber or vitamin B and are very high-glycemic foods. These could cause spikes in your blood sugar and makes your body store fat.

- Caffeine

Have you ever stopped to think about what goes into your body when you sip coffee or drink that energy drink? Caffeine, just like alcohol, gets into the bloodstream fast and it will take 45 minutes for about 99 percent of the caffeine to get absorbed through the membranes of the stomach, throat, and mouth. Caffeine is considered basic but cola, hot chocolate, energy drinks, tea, and coffee are acid-forming because there are other chemicals in play like acetic acid, formic acid, and phosphorus. Once it has been absorbed, the liver will metabolize caffeine and the by-products get filtered by the kidneys and leave the body through urine. To lessen the stress on your liver, try to switch your normal coffee for herbal tea or a glass of water.

- Refined sugar

Americans consume way too much sugar, and just like sodium, it is found in most of the foods we eat. A normal American will consume around 22 teaspoons of sugar daily. This can add up to more than 70 pounds each year. The current recommendation for adding sugar is no more than five teaspoons daily for women and between eight and nine teaspoons daily for men. Consuming too much sugar could lead to high cholesterol, diabetes, high blood sugar, and unhealthy weight gain. The biggest sources of added sugars are foods like dairy, desserts, cookies, cakes, candy, and soft drinks. Look at the nutrition label on foods to find out how much sugar is in the foods you consume daily. Fresh whole foods don't contain added sugar; try to stick with eating natural foods that contain nutrient-rich sugars the way nature intended it to be.

- Animal products

The highest acid-forming foods you eat are found in dairy, eggs, and meat. In the United States, people eat way too much animal products. They make it the center point of the meal instead of using it as a side. Animal proteins, if they aren't organic, could contain antibiotics and hormones. Animal proteins are high in cholesterol and saturated fats. Eggs and meat contain many sulfur-containing amino acids that get metabolized into sulfuric acid and has to be buffered by the body by using calcium compounds and this puts more strain on the kidneys. Your body has to have sufficient protein to recover and repair the body, so you can't get rid of protein entirely. You need to balance out your choices and use ones that are alkaline-forming. With the alkaline diet, you are going to get a lot of nutrient-rich, fiber-packed plant proteins by swapping meat for legumes and beans a couple times each week.

Foods to Enjoy

Good news is that there isn't a shortage of alkalizing foods that feed our bodies with lots of antioxidants, phytochemicals, minerals, and vitamins that will improve your health and add vitality. Use the following foods to find all the health benefits for the foods that are allowed on this diet. Focus on the foods you can add instead of what you should get rid of or reduce. Making a subtle shift in the way you think can make a huge difference. It can remove judgment, anxiety, and stress. Eat the good foods first and you might realize there isn't any room left for bad stuff.

- Nightshades – PRAL -8.6

Members of the common nightshade family include hot chili peppers, sweet bell peppers, tomatoes, eggplant, white potatoes, and any spice that is made from peppers like

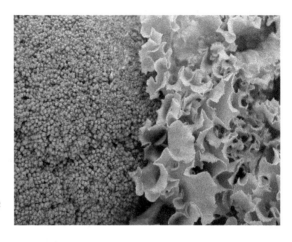

cayenne pepper, red pepper flakes, and paprika. This is a small list but it contains a large number of important benefits. Tomatoes are a good source of lycopene which is a phytochemical. This can lower your risk of developing prostate cancer. Capsaicin, which is a compound found in peppers, is a powerful anti-inflammatory for the body. All these foods are high in fiber, vitamin C, and other minerals including magnesium and potassium.

- Eggplant – PRAL -3.4

Besides the fact that it is alkaline, eggplants is a food that offers phytonutrients like chlorogenic acid. This acid is not acidifying to the body, instead, it is a plant compound that helps aid your metabolism and digestion. Eggplants are also delicious when you bake it in some olive oil, added to salads, or used as a pizza crust.

- Pears – PRAL -2.9

Pears have high fiber content and low sugar content, which is a great fruit even for people who suffer from blood sugar imbalances. Pears also have a lot of vitamin C content, which is great for protecting your cells from carcinogens.

- Beet Greens – PRAL -16.7

Let's hear it for the most alkaline food in the world: beet greens. While beet greens may not be one of the most popular greens in our currently diet, their amazing alkalinity score makes them a great choice to add into stir-fries or smoothies. Besides the fact that they have a high alkaline content, beet greens are also slightly bitter that could end up helping stimulate bile productions in order to help you digest fats better.

If this doesn't give you enough of a reason to stops throwing out your beet tops, I don't know what will. Beet greens can be used to replace any type of greens you use in smoothies, soups, or salads.

- Hazelnuts – PRAL -2.8

The majority of nuts come with an acidifying effect, but hazelnuts have proven to be the exception to the rule. So if you enjoy nuts, these are the best choice to include into your daily diet in comparison to peanuts, which have a score of +8 and are highly acidic to your body. Hazelnuts are famous for their contribution to nut butters, such as Nutella, but your make your own version of this that is healthy if you enjoy this particular spread.

- Pineapple – PRAL -2.7

Pineapple is very alkalizing and delicious, plus they are good for your digestion, so much so, several dietary supplements add them to digestive-boosting formulas. This is due to the fact that pineapples contain a digestive enzyme known as bromelain. Bromelain is also believed to be helpful in killing of intestinal parasites.

- Leafy greens – PRAL -11.8

Leafy green vegetables are the most nutritious foods that you could eat. It doesn't matter if you put them into a smoothie or eat them as a salad; these are very alkalizing and high in phytochemicals and nutrients. Yes, all greens are nutritious, but some of the top choices for maximum health include mustard greens, arugula, turnip greens, Swiss chard, spinach, and kale. Greens are nutritional powerhouses and are high in fiber. They don't have many calories and contain lots of vitamin K and calcium for bone health. Greens are also high in vitamins C and A, potassium, along with zeaxanthin and lutein. Studies show that the phytochemicals and carotenoids in folate greens might help reduce the risk of certain cancers, helps with managing weight, and lowers the chance of type 2 polygenic disease.

Spinach, specifically, is also for its bone health properties because of its calcium content. Because it is highly alkalizing, anti-cancer juicing protocols will often include spinach into their regimen.

- Kale – PRAL -8.3

People don't refer kale as the new beef for nothing. Kale is high in vitamin K, calcium, and iron, which is believed to be a great protector against many forms of cancer. Besides all of these benefits, kale is another extremely alkaline food. Kale is mild in taste and you can add it into any recipes to help jazz it up. Kale can easily be added into recipes that call for greens, or in soups, salads and stir fires.

- Swiss Chard – PRAL -8.1

Have you started to see a trend here? Some of the world's most alkaline foods are leafy greens. Swiss chard is just another green that can provide you with a whole lot of nutritious benefits with vitamins that help to support our cellular health, like vitamin K. Swiss chard also has plant protein and phosphorus, but the PRAL score tells us that it leaves behind more alkalizing minerals than it does acidity when the body metabolizes it. Swiss chard is great to use as the wrap for a lettuce wrap in any recipe that calls for a tortilla or any sort of grain bread.

- Squashes – PRAL -8.6 to -6.0

Squash is an umbrella term that covers many types of vegetables that include winter squashes like cushaw, butternut, Hubbard, and acorn, summer varieties like crookneck and zucchini, and pumpkins. Squash is very versatile and can be substituted for noodles, julienned, or put into stir-fries or salads. Squashes are high in vitamin A, E, B, and C along with the minerals iron, calcium, potassium, and magnesium. Adding squash into your diet could keep your heart healthy due to the potassium. It also lowers inflammation by providing the phytochemicals beta-carotene, zeaxanthin, and lutein. It protects against certain cancers by adding carotenoids and vitamin A.

- Bananas – PRAL -6.9

Bananas, or as I like to call them, potassium sticks, are another great food to eat that is highly alkalizing, plus, it's also delicious. Bananas are a perfect source of fiber, which will help to promote your digestive regularity and get rid of any toxins within your gastrointestinal tract. You eat enough bananas; your colon won't be missing those grains. While a lot of people want to stay away from bananas when they are trying to lose weight because of their sugar content, eating a banana is a lot better for you than grabbing a handful of granola or some other pre-packaged processed food that is full of unhealthy sugars and acidifying ingredients.

One of the best ways you can add more bananas to your diet is to use it to make ice cream. All you have to do is freeze peeled bananas and then blend them up until they form a creamy consistency. The part is that you can add in other alkalizing foods to change up the flavor, like berries and mint.

- Zucchini – PRAL -2.6

Zucchini contains lutein, which is a great source of phytonutrients. Lutein is part of the same category of antioxidants as beta-carotene, which means that it can help with eye health. Zucchini has carved itself a niche in the diet world as being a vegan, gluten-free, low-carb pasta alternative. A spiralizer can be used to make zucchini pasta noodles, know lovingly as zoodles. Toss them in your favorite alkaline pasta sauce, and you have a delicious meal.

- Strawberries – PRAL -2.2

Strawberries are another great source of vitamin C. They also have a high manganese contain, which is a trace mineral that the body needs to help facilitate metabolic function. There are an endless number of ways to enjoy strawberries.

- Apples – PRAL -2.2

Apples have long been viewed as one of the healthiest foods in the world, mainly because they have a high content of detoxifying fiber and vitamin C, as well as flavonoids that help to fight off cancer. These are all essential nutrients for the body and help to promote healthy cholesterol and blood pressure levels. To get even more health benefits from these delicious foods, it's a good idea to add apple cider vinegar to your daily diet. When apples are fermented to make vinegar, they contain a nutrient known as acetic acid, which provides antiviral and antibacterial benefits. If you're not a fan of the taste of apple cider vinegar, whether diluted or not, that's fine, there are many other ways you can use apple cider vinegar without having to taste it.

- Lentils and beans – PRAL -14.4 to 8.6

Legumes and beans are full of nutritious things. Packed in each bean is potassium, iron, B vitamins, fiber, little to no sodium or fat, and plant proteins that are heart healthy. Beans can lower the risk for cancer and heart disease because all the many different phytochemicals that are present. Beans lower cholesterol because they give the body soluble fiber. This is the

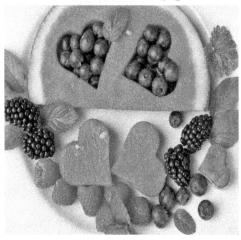

same fiber that helps you feel full and keeps your glucose steady. Some choices in this group are acidic but they aren't as acidifying as animal proteins. The best beans to choose are yellow and green like split peas, lima beans, pigeon peas, black beans, and kidney beans.

- Watermelon – PRAL -1.9

Watermelon is another healthy alkalizing food that can help to provide you body with important electrolytes to aid in cardiac function, like potassium. Since watermelons are made up of mostly water, they also keep you hydrated more so than any other vegetables and fruits. Watermelon is a delicious snack, but you can also have fun and get creative with it.

- Crucifers – PRAL -1.2 to -4.9

This is the most nutritious group of foods. When talking about nutrients, their states are extremely high in vitamins C and A, fiber, folic acid, and carotenoids. Collards and kale are technically leafy greens but are cruciferous vegetables and contain more vitamin K than all other vegetables. The phytochemical content of these vegetables can lower the risk of developing certain cancers including breast, lung, colorectal, and prostate. They are low in calories and are alkaline-forming. In order to get all their benefits, try to consume one to two cups each day. There is a lot to choose from such as cauliflower, bok choy, kale, collard greens, cabbage, Brussels sprouts, and broccoli.

Cauliflower is an amazing alkaline food that can help to aid in rebalancing your hormones when the estrogen levels in your body are too high. This is due to the fact that cauliflower contains what is call Indole-3-Carbinol, which helps your body to regular estrogen levels. We all come in contact with estrogen regularly through foods that contain estrogen, like soy, chemicals within our environment, like plastics, and pharmaceutical drugs, like oral contraceptives. Too much estrogen within then body is very harmful to the body and can cause digestive problems like bloating, weight gain, and can cause infertility and reproductive cancers.

- Cherries – PRAL -3.6

Cherries have already made a name for themselves as one of the best sources of antioxidants like anthocyanins, which help to reduce your cancer risk. Studies have also found that cherries are great at relieving inflammation linked to arthritis and joint pain, and could even help to prevent cardiovascular disease. Cherries can easily be added to smoothies. When you have a post-workout shake, you want to make sure it includes plenty of alkaline foods. This is due to the fact that lactic acid, which is a substance that naturally helps to improve your body's energy, is released naturally during an intense exercise. As you can guess by its name, lactic acid will make the body more acidic, which is the reason for consuming alkaline foods after a workout to help neutralize the acids.

- Seeds and nuts – PRAL -1.4

For some people, some of their favorite nuts could be moderately acid-forming like pecans, peanuts, hazelnuts, and walnuts. There are still a lot of varieties of seeds and nuts you can eat that will have alkalizing effects on the body. Chestnuts are among the most alkaline-forming nut because of their water content. The next is almonds that are second on the alkaline scale. Nuts, even the ones that are slightly acidic still contain vitamin E, zinc, magnesium, fiber, and healthy fats. Seeds that you can eat while following the alkaline diet include sunflower, sesame, flax, hemp, and chia. Adding nuts as a part of your healthy diet can bring benefits to your heart, add nutrients, and help weight management by making you feel fuller longer.

- Celery – PRAL -5.2

Aside from the fact that it is alkalizing, celery also comes along with some cleansing properties. Since it is made up of mostly water, celery is able to flush toxins from the body. Celery is also one of those magic "negative calorie" foods. This means that when you eat celery, it will require your body to burn more calories to chew and digest it than it actually contains. Celery is a great addition to smoothie and juice recipes.

- Carrots – PRAL -4.9

Carrots are another great alkaline food and they are also famous for improving eyesight due to their vitamin A content. Just a single cup of carrots has more than 300% of the recommended daily intake of beta-carotene, which is the antioxidant form of vitamin A. Beta-carotene also has the ability to protect against cancer and it helps your skin to look younger and brighter.

- Kiwi – PRAL -4.1

Kiwi is another delicious fruit that is highly alkalizing. It contains a plethora of minerals, vitamins, and antioxidants. While oranges have long been the kind of vitamin C, kiwi fruit contains almost five times the amount of vitamin C than an orange does. Kiwi also provides your body with fiber to help improve your digestion, and it contains potassium, which helps with muscle function.

- Tubers – PRAL -5.6

While you are working on trying to decrease the grains you eat, you might be asking what in the world can I eat to fill in this void. This answer is simple, tubers. Tubers are plants that develop starchy roots and are foods from ancient civilizations. They have been prized for their wonderful benefits. They are considered complex carbs, tubers give our bodies blood sugar. They provide stabilizing slow-burning energy. They are high in antioxidants, magnesium, potassium, vitamins C and A, phytochemicals, and fiber. Tubers can help lower the risk of heart disease, lowers the risk of cancer, and keeps your bones healthy. Tubers are a low-calorie option to be used in place of other starchy, grain-based carbs. Your best bet is cassava, yams, and sweet potatoes.

You don't have to feel guilty about your love for sweet potatoes fires. While they may be a starchy vegetable, sweet potatoes are amazingly alkalizing, and it provides your body with lots of minerals, vitamins, and fiber. Since sweet potatoes have a high fiber content, they don't have as much of an impact on your blood sugar levels, since the fiber content works to slow down the release of sugar to your bloodstream. Therefore, sweet potatoes are a great food to consume when you need some energy and some alkalinity.

Recipes

Breakfast

Hemp Seed and Carrot Muffins

Serves: 12
Cashew butter, 6 tbsp
Shredded carrot,
Unrefined whole cane sugar, .5 c.
Almond milk, 1 c.
Oat flour, 2 c.
Ground flaxseed, 1 tbsp
Water, 3 tbsp
Pinch of sea salt
Vanilla bean powder, pinch
Baking powder, 1 tbsp
Chopped kale, 1 tbsp
Hemp seeds, 2 tbsp

1. Start by placing your oven to 350.

2. Beat the flaxseed and water together to make the flax egg.

3. Pour this into a bigger bowl then combine within the salt, vanilla bean-flavored powder, baking powder, kale, hemp seeds, cashew butter, carrot, sugar, almond milk, and oat flour. Stir everything together until well combined.

4. Grease a 12-cup muffin tin and divide the batter between the cups. Bake for 20-25 minutes and enjoy.

Chia Seed and Strawberry Parfait

Serves: 2

Strawberry Mixture –

Brown rice syrup, 1-2 tsp

Chia seeds, 1 tsp

Diced strawberries, 1 c.

Oat Mixture –

Quick rolled oats, 1 c.

Vanilla bean powder, pinch

Brown rice syrup, 1 tbsp

Coconut milk, 1 c.

1. To make the strawberry mixture, stir together the brown rice syrup, chia seeds, and strawberries in a small bowl until well-mixed.

2. In a separate bowl, mix together the vanilla bean powder, brown rice syrup, coconut milk, and oats until well-mixed.

3. Place portion of the oats in the base of two small jars. Cover with a portion of the strawberry mixture. Repeat this with the remaining ingredients.

4. Put a cover on the jars and let them to refrigerate all night long.

5. The next morning, uncover and enjoy.

Pecan Pancakes

Serves: 5

Chopped pecans, .25 c.

Nutmeg, .25 tsp

Cinnamon, .5 tsp

Vanilla, 1 tsp

Melted butter, 2 tbsp

Unsweetened soy milk, .75 c.

Eggs, 2

Salt, .25 tsp

Baking powder, .25 tsp

Granular sugar substitute, 1 tbsp

Almond flour, .75 c.

Olive oil - cooking spray

1. Place the salt, sugar substitute, baking powder, and almond flour into a bowl and mix well.

2. In another bowl, put the vanilla, soy milk, butter, and eggs. Mix well to incorporate everything.

3. Place the egg mixture into the dried-up contents and mix well till well-blended.

4. Add nutmeg, pecans, and cinnamon. Stir for five minutes.

5. Place a twelve-inch cooking pan onto average hot temperature and sprinkle by using cookery spray.

6. Scoop one tablespoon of batter into the preheated skillet and spread out into a four-inch circle.

7. Place three more spoonfuls into the skillet and cook until bubbles have formed at the edges of the pancakes and the bottoms are browned.

8. Flip each one and cook another two minutes.

9. Repeat the process until all batter has been used.

10. Serve with syrup of choice.

Quinoa Breakfast

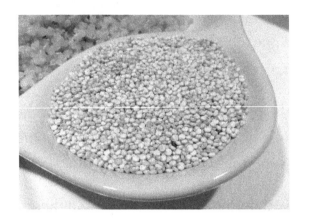

Serves: 4

Maple syrup, 3 tbsp

2-inch cinnamon stick

Water, 2 c.

Quinoa, 1 c.

Optional Toppings:

Yogurt

Chopped cashew, 2 tbsp

Whipped coconut cream, 3 tbsp

Lime juice, 1 tsp

Nutmeg, .25 tsp

Raisins, 2 tbsp

Strawberries, .5 c.

Raspberries, .5 c.

Blueberries, .5 c.

1. Put the quinoa into a strainer and rinse it under cold running water. Make sure there aren't any stones or anything in them.

2. Pour water into a saucepan. Add the quinoa and place saucepan on medium heat. Bring to a boil.

3. Add in the cinnamon stick, place a cover on the saucepan, lower hot temperature, also, boil gently quarter-hour till water has been ingested.

4. Take off hot temperature and fluff with a fork. Add maple syrup and any of the toppings listed above.

Oatmeal

Serves: 4

Salt

Steel-cut oats, 1.25 c.

Water, 3.75 c.

Optional Toppings:

Nuts

Dried fruits

Sliced banana

Diced mangoes

Mixed berries

Garam masala, 1 tsp

Lemon pepper, .25 tsp

Nutmeg, .25 tsp

Cinnamon, 1 tsp

1. Place a saucepan on medium and add water. Let the water boil.

2. Pour in the oats along with a dash of salt and lower the heat to a simmer.

3. Let simmer 25 minutes, stirring constantly.

4. Once all the water has been absorbed, add in any of the toppings listed above if you want to add in any flavor. If you want it creamier, add in a tablespoon of coconut milk.

Baked Grapefruit

Serves: 1

Unsweetened grated coconut, 2 tbsp

Halved grapefruit, 1

1. You need to warm your oven to 350.

2. Take some foil and line a baking sheet with it.

3. Place the halved grapefruit cut side up on the foil. Top each with one tablespoon of coconut.

4. Put into broiler and prepare quarter-hour or till coconut is tanned.

5. Carefully remove from oven and enjoy.

Almond Pancakes

Serves: 4

Coconut oil, 3 tbsp

Almond milk, 1 c.

Baking powder, 1 tsp

Arrowroot powder, 2 tbsp

Almond flour, 1 c.

1. Place each of the dry fixings in a dish and whip to mix.

2. Add two tablespoons of coconut oil together with almond milk to the dry fixings and blend well till everything is all around blended.

3. Place a skillet on medium and put one teaspoon coconut in it to melt. Swirl it around in the skillet to coat.

4. Pour one ladle of batter into the skillet and using the bottom of the ladle to smooth out pancake.

5. Cook for three minutes until edges are bubbly and brown.

6. Flip pancake and cook another three minutes until cooked through.

7. Continue cooking pancakes until all batter is used.

Amaranth Porridge

Serves: 2

Cinnamon, 1 tbsp

Coconut oil, 2 tbsp

Amaranth, 1 c.

Alkaline water, 2 c.

Almond milk, 2 c.

1. Flow the water together with the milk into a pot. Place on medium hot temperature and allow to boil.

2. Stir in amaranth and turn down the hot temperature to a low level. Stew for half an hour mixing every now and then.

3. Take off hot temperature, add in copra oil and cinnamon, stir well, serve warm.

Banana Porridge

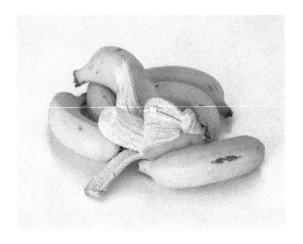

Serves: 2

Chopped almonds, .25 c.

Liquid stevia, 3 drops

Barley, .5 c.

Sliced banana, 1

Unsweetened almond milk, 1 c.

1. Mix the stevia, one half cup almond milk, and barley in a bowl.

2. Place in the refrigerator, covered for six hours.

3. Take out of the refrigerator and mix in the remaining milk. Pour into a saucepan and place on medium. Allow mixture to cook for five minutes.

Zucchini Muffins

Serves: 16

Salt

Cinnamon, 1 tsp

Baking powder, 1 tbsp

Almond flour, 2 c.

Vanilla extract, 1 tsp

Almond milk, .5 c.

Grated zucchinis, 2

Overripe bananas, 3

Almond butter, .25 c.

Alkaline water, 3 tbsp

Ground flaxseed, 1 tbsp

Optional Ingredients:

Chopped walnuts, .25 c.

Chocolate chips, .25 c.

1. You need to warm your kitchen appliance to 375 degrees. Sprinkle a cupcake tin by using cookery spray.

2. Place the water and flaxseed in a bowl.

3. Mash the bananas in a pot and put in altogether the leftover contents. Blend nicely.

4. Separate concoction evenly in a cupcake tin.

5. Place into the oven for 25 minutes.

Vegetable Tofu Scramble

Serves: 4

Salt

Chopped basil, 2 tbsp

Chopped firm tofu, 3 c.

Diced peppers (red, bell), 2 pcs.

Olive oil, 1 tablespoon

Turmeric

Chopped cherry tomatoes, 2 c.

Chopped onions, 2

Cayenne

1. Place a greased skillet on medium and warm the pan.

2. Put on bell peppers together with onions, prepare for five minutes.

3. Put in tofu, cayenne, salt, and turmeric. Cook an additional eight minutes.

4. Garnish with basil.

Zucchini Pancakes

Serves: 8

Finely chopped scallions, .5 c.

Finely chopped jalapeno, 2

Olive oil, 2 tsp

Ground flax seeds, 4 tbsp

Salt

Grated zucchini, 6

Alkaline water, 12 tbsp

1. Place the flax seeds and water into a bowl and mix well. Sit to the side.

2. Place a large skillet on medium and warm oil. Add on pepper, salt, and zucchini. Cook three minutes and place zucchini in a bowl.

3. Add in flaxseed mixture and scallions and mix well.

4. Warm a griddle that has been sprayed with cooking spray. Pour some zucchini onto the preheated griddle and cook three minutes per side until golden.

5. Repeat until mixture is completely used up.

Pumpkin Quinoa

Serves: 2

Chia seeds, 2 teaspoons

Pumpkin pie spice, 1 teaspoon

Pumpkin puree, .25 c.

Mashed banana, 1

Unsweetened almond milk, 1 c.

Cooked quinoa, 1 c.

1. Put all ingredients into a container.

2. Make sure the lid is sealed and shake well to combine.

3. Place in the refrigerator overnight.

4. When ready to eat, take out of the fridge and enjoy.

Avocado Toast

Serves: 4

Dulse flakes, sliced radish, sliced red onion, for topping – optional

Sea salt, .5 tsp

Fresh cilantro leaves, 1 tbsp

Chopped onion, 1 tbsp

Garlic, 2 cloves

Jalapeno

Avocado, 2

Unpeeled sweet potato, sliced into 4 thick lengthwise slices

1. Lay each of the slices of potato in a toaster slot and toast them for four cycles, or until they are cooked through. You can also toast them in the oven if you don't have a regular toaster. You want them to get tender enough to be pierced easily with a fork. Carefully place the cooked "toast" on plates.

2. Since the sweet potato toast cooks, add the salt, cilantro, onion, garlic, jalapeno, and avocado in an exceedingly electric kitchen appliance and blend till it becomes creamy and smooth. Adjust the amount of salt you use as needed.

3. Divide the avocado spread over the top each of the sweet potato toast slices. Top each with your desired toppings of choice. Enjoy.

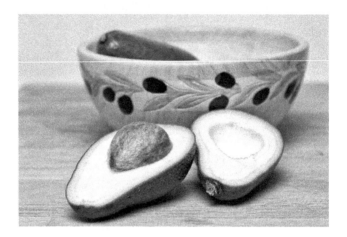

Frozen Banana Breakfast Bowl

Serves: 1

Chia seeds, hemp seeds, unsweetened coconut flakes, for topping – optional

Pumpkin seed protein powder, 4 tbsp

Bananas, 2

1. Peel and then slice the bananas. Place thin in a freezer-safe container and freeze them overnight.

2. The next morning, add the bananas to a food processor and mix until they reach a creamy and smooth consistency, much like soft-serve ice cream.

3. Process the pumpkin protein powder through the bananas until just combined.

4. Pour into a serving dish and top with your desired toppings if you so choose to and enjoy.

Chia Seed and Blueberry Cobbler

Serves: 4

Blueberry Mixture –

Chia seeds, 1 tbsp

Unrefined whole cane sugar, 2 tbsp

Blueberries, 2 c.

Topping –

Almond flour, .5 c.

Sea salt, .25 teaspoon

Vanilla bean powder, 1 teaspoon

A mixture of Sodium Bicarbonate and cream of tartar, 1.5 teaspoon

Unrefined whole cane sugar, 2 tablespoons

Melted coconut oil, 2 tablespoons

Coconut milk, 4 tablespoons

Oat flour, .5 c.

1. Start by placing your oven to 350.

2. To get the blueberries ready, mix the chia seeds, sugar, and blueberries together. Place the blueberry mixture into the bottom of four 4-ounce ovenproof ramekins.

3. To fix the topping, mix together the salt, vanilla bean powder, baking powder, sugar, coconut oil, coconut milk, oat flour, and almond flour.

4. Divide the topping over the blueberries in the four ramekins. You can either leave the topping as dollops, or you can spread them out evenly over the blueberry mixture to create a full crust.

5. Bake the cobblers for 45 minutes, or until the topping has turned golden and everything is heated through. Enjoy.

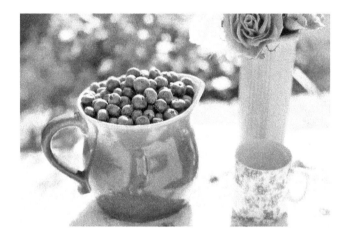

Quick and Easy Granola Bars

Serves: 6

Vanilla bean powder, .25 teaspoon

Cinnamon spice, .25 teaspoon

Seawater salt, .25 teaspoon

Coconut oil, 1 tablespoon

Brown rice syrup, 2 tablespoons

Almond butter, .5 c.

Quick rolled oats, 1 c.

1. Place some parchment into the bottom of a 9x5 inch loaf pan.

2. Add the vanilla bean powder, cinnamon, salt, coconut oil, brown rice syrup, almond butter, and oats to a food processor and mix until they are well-combined.

3. Run the concoction into the loaf frying pan as well as push it down into an even mixture, ensure that it's well-compressed. Refrigerate the bars for 15 to 20 minutes, or until they are completely firm.

4. Slice the granola into six bars and enjoy. Keep any leftovers in the refrigerator. At room temp, they will become soft.

Lunch

Roasted Artichoke Salad

Serves: 2

Paprika, pinch

Garlic powder, pinch

Pepper, pinch

Sea salt, pinch

Avocado oil, 1 tbsp

Drained artichoke hearts, 14 oz

Mixed salad greens, 2-4 c.

Dressing –

Pepper, pinch

Sea salt, pinch

Diced shallot

Brown rice sweetening, 1 tablespoon

Sesame pits, 1 tablespoon

Apple vinegar, 2 tablespoons

Avocado oil, 2 tbsp

1. Start by placing your oven to 425. Place some parchment on a baking sheet.

2. Slice the tips off of the artichokes and then slice the hearts in half. Rub them with some oil.

3. Mix together the paprika, garlic, pepper, and salt. Lay the artichokes on the baking sheet and sprinkle them with the seasoning mixture. Toss everything to coat.

4. Roast them for 30 minutes, tossing again halfway through the cooking time.

5. As the artichokes roast, beat together the pepper, salt, shallot, brown rice syrup, sesame seeds, vinegar, and avocado oil. Make sure everything is well mixed. Adjust any of the flavors as you need.

6. To assemble the salad, toss the mixed salad greens with the artichokes and then drizzle on the dressing. Divide into two plates and enjoy.

Sunchoke Hash

Serves: 4

Sliced scallion

EVOO

Pepper

Salt

Thinly sliced Brussels sprouts, 6

Sliced sunchokes, 4

1. Pour some cold water into a bowl.

2. Place the sliced sunchokes into the water and let them sit.

3. Rinse thoroughly and dry using paper towels.

4. Place a pan on medium and warm up some EVOO.

5. Add the sunchokes and Brussels sprouts. Cook for four minutes.

6. Sprinkle with pepper and salt.

7. Serve with a drizzle of olive oil and sprinkle on the sliced scallions.

Vegetable Fritters

Serves: 2

Cooking spray

Water, .25 c.

Garlic powder, .5 tsp

Salt, 1 tsp

Almond flour, .25 c.

Scallions, 4

Grated onion, .5

Chopped yellow squash, 1

Peeled and chopped carrot, 1

Chopped zucchini, 1

1. Place the scallion, almond flour, yellow squash, zucchini, carrot, garlic powder, and salt into a food processor.

2. Pulse until everything is thoroughly blended.

3. Add just enough water to make sure mixture is moist and thick.

4. Place an oversized pan on standard heat and sprinkle by using preparation spray.

5. When the oil is heated, use an ice cream scoop and add put mixture into skillet. Cook for three minutes each side.

6. Use back of ice cream scoop to spread the mixture around.

Mint Lime Salad

Serves: 4

Lemon juice, 2 tbsp

Chopped mint, 2 tbsp

Strawberries, .25 c.

Diced Peaches, .25 c.

Tangerine segments, .25 c.

Bite-size cantaloupe pieces, .25 c.

Bite-size honeydew pieces, .25 c.

Bite-size watermelon pieces, .25 c.

Diced apple, .25 c.

Grapes, .25 c.

1. Put all fruits into a bowl. Add in mint and lemon juice.

2. Mix well and cover.

3. Place in the refrigerator and chill overnight.

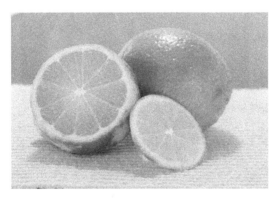

Zucchini Salad

Serves: 2

Fresh herbs of choice, 1 tsp

Pepper

Salt

EVOO, 2 tbsp

Juice of .5 lemon

Minced garlic, 1 clove

Sliced onion, 1

Diced tomato, 2

Red bell pepper, 1

Sliced zucchini, 1

4. Wash all vegetables and set to the side.

5. Cut the ends off the zucchini. Cut in half lengthwise and then slice into half-moons.

6. Dice the tomatoes.

7. Cut the bell pepper in half, clean out the ribs and seeds and slice each half.

8. Cut the top and bottom off the onion and remove outer peel. Thinly slice into rings.

9. Add all the prepared vegetables into a bowl.

10. In a separate bowl add pepper, salt, herbs, olive oil, garlic, and lemon juice. Mix well to combine.

11. Pour over vegetables and toss to coat.

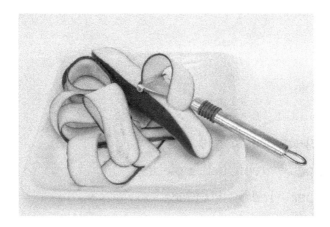

Stir Fried Tofu

Serves: 4

Fresh herbs

Ginger, .25 tbsp

Curry powder, .5 tbsp

Pepper

Salt

EVOO, 2 tbsp

Coconut milk, 1.5 c.

Chopped green beans, .5 lb.

Diced pepper – green, bell, 1 piece

Diced pepper – red, bell, 1 piece

Diced tomatoes, 3

Chopped zucchinis, 3

Diced firm tofu, 1 lb.

1. Place a saucepan on medium, warm oil. Add in tofu and cook about three minutes.

2. Add in zucchini, beans, and bell peppers. Stir fry for an additional three minutes.

3. Add tomatoes and coconut milk and stir well. Let it simmer for a little more time.

4. Season with herbs, curry powder, pepper, salt, and ginger.

5. Serve with wild rice.

Potato Pumpkin Patties

Serves: 2

EVOO

Pepper

Salt

Chopped parsley, 3 tbsp

Water, 4 tbsp

Soy flour, 2.5 oz

Potatoes, 1 lb.

Pumpkin, 1 lb.

1. Peel the potatoes and pumpkin. Cut them into large chunks.

2. Place into a food processor and process until small pieces but not mush.

3. Add the water and soy flour to a bowl. Mix well.

4. Take the pumpkin and potato out of the food processor and place them into a different bowl.

5. Pour on the flour mixture and mix well.

6. Season with pepper, parsley, and salt.

7. Place a skillet on medium and warm up some EVOO.

8. Turn the potato and pumpkin mixture into patties. Place prepared patties into the skillet and fry for three minutes per side.

Italian Stir-Fry

Serves: 2

Water, .5 c

Pepper

Curry powder, .5 teaspoon

Oregano plant, 1 teaspoon

Parsley, one tablespoon

Sodium Chloride, 1 teaspoon

Grated cheddar, 1 tbsp

EVOO, 2 tbsp

Diced tomatoes, 2

Slivered zucchini, 1

Diced onion, 2

Slivered leeks, 2

1. Take a skillet and place on medium warm up the olive oil.

2. Put the onions into the skillet and cook until soft.

3. Add zucchini and cook another four minutes. Pour water into the skillet and place a lid on it.

4. Lower heat and simmer for ten minutes.

5. Carefully remove the lid and add tomatoes. Season with curry powder and pepper. Replace lid and cook an additional ten minutes.

6. When cooked through, taste and adjust seasonings if needed.

7. Sprinkle with cheese and serve with bread if your diet allows it.

Southern Salad

Serves: 4

Salsa, .5 c.

Cilantro, .5 c.

Chopped almonds, .25 c.

Diced avocado, 1

Halved cherry tomatoes, 1 c.

Sprouted black beans, .5 c.

Romaine lettuce, 5 c.

1. Put each of the contents into an oversized bowl then throw nicely.

2. Divide into salad bowls and serve.

Roasted Vegetables

Serves: 4

Salt

Alliaceous (garlic) powder, 1 tablespoon

Coconut oil, 1 tablespoon

Pepper – chopped, bell – yellow, one

Pepper – chopped, bell - red, one

Chopped carrot, one

Trimmed asparagus, .5 bunch

Cherry tomatoes, 1 pint

Halved mushrooms, .5 c.

1. You need to warm your oven to 425.

2. Place the carrot, bell peppers, tomatoes, mushrooms, and asparagus into a large bowl.

3. In another basin, put in the garlic powder, Sodium Chloride, together with coconut milk. Blend nicely.

4. Run over the vegetables and toss to coat.

5. Pour vegetables onto a cooking film then place in the stove for 15 minutes till veggies are tender.

6. Divide onto four plates and enjoy.

Pad Thai Salad

Serves: 2

Salt, .5 tsp

Stevia, 1 packet

Tamarind paste, 1 tsp

Minced garlic, 1 clove

Juice of one lime

Chopped almonds, 2 tbsp

Chopped scallions, 1

Stripped zucchini, 1

Thinly sliced carrot, 2

Bean sprouts, 1 c.

Iceberg lettuce, 4 c.

1. Place the almonds, bean sprouts, zucchini, carrots, and lettuce into a large bowl.

2. Place the salt, stevia, lime juice, tamarind paste, and garlic into a small food processor. Process until well blended.

3. Pour dressing over the vegetables and toss to coat.

4. Evenly divide into serving bowls.

Cucumber Salad

Serves: 4

Pepper

Salt

Sesame seed oil, 3 tbsp

Minced garlic, 4 cloves

Cucumber, 1 lb.

1. Place the pepper, salt, sesame seed oil, and garlic to a bowl. Whisk well to combine.

2. Wash cucumbers and cut the ends off. Cut them in half lengthwise and then slice into half-moons.

3. Add to dressing mixture to the cucumbers and toss well to coat.

4. Place in the refrigerator for ten minutes. Enjoy.

Red Lentil Pasta Salad

Serves: 4

For the Dressing and Pasta –

Pepper, .25 tsp

Sea salt, .25 tsp

Dried oregano, 1 tsp

Juice - Lemon, one tablespoon

Apple vinegar, two tablespoons

Avocado - oil, .25 c.

Red lentil pasta, 2 c.

Veggies –

Crushed garlic, 2 cloves

Sliced summer squash, .5

Sliced zucchini, .5

Diced red onion, .33 c.

Chopped pepper – orange, bell, 1 c.

Chopped asparagus stalks, 6

Avocado oil, 1 tbsp

1. Cook the pasta following the directions on the package.

2. As the pasta is cooking, whisk the pepper, salt, oregano, lemon juice, vinegar, and avocado oil together until well combined. Adjust any of the seasonings that you need to.

3. For the veggies, warm the oil in an exceedingly frying pan then cook the garlic bulb, squash, zucchini, onion, bell pepper, and asparagus. Cook for two to three minutes, or until they are soft.

4. Add the pasta, veggies, and dressing in a bowl and toss everything together. Divide into four plates and enjoy.

Peach Salsa Salad

Serves: 2

Dressing –

Pinch sea salt

Lemon juice, 1 tsp

Water, .25 c

Brown rice syrup, 3 to 4 tbsp

Tahini, 4 tbsp

Salsa –

Diced jalapeno, .5

Chopped purple onion, one tablespoon

Diced coriander, one tablespoon

Chopped pepper – red, bell, .25 c.

Cubed and pitted peach

Assembling –

Mixed salad greens – 3 c

1. For the dressing, whisk together the salt, lemon juice, water, brown rice syrup, and tahini until combined. Adjust any of the seasonings that you need to.

2. Throw each of the condiment ingredients along inside another container.

3. To make the salad, place the salad greens on two plates and top with the salsa. Drizzle on the dressing and enjoy.

Pineapple Salad

Serves: 1

Dressing –

Chopped cilantro, .5 c.

Chopped scallions, .5 c.

Lime juice, 2 tbsp

Water, .25 c.

Avocado oil, .25 c.

Sea salt, .5 tsp

Garlic, 2 cloves

Assembling –

Dulse flakes

Chopped purple cabbage, 1 c.

Cubed pineapple, .5 c.

Mixed salad greens, 2 c.

1. Put each of the dressing contents to your liquidizer then blend till nicely combined. Adjust any of the seasonings that you need to.

2. To make your salad, add the salad green to a bowl and top with the dulse flakes, purple cabbage, and pineapple. Drizzle on the dressing and toss together. Enjoy.

Sweet Potato Salad with Jalapeno Dressing

Serves: 2

Sweet Potatoes –

Sea salt, .25 tsp

Paprika, 1 tsp

Crushed garlic, 2 cloves

Avocado oil, 2 tbsp

Peeled and cubed sweet potatoes, 3

Dressing –

Water, 1 c.

Sea salt, .5 tsp

Lime juice, 2 tbsp

Jalapeno

Cilantro leaves, .25 c.

Raw cashews, 1 c.

Assembling –

Mixed salad greens, 2 c.

1. Start by placing your kitchen appliance to three hundred and fifty degrees. Put some parchment on a cooking film.

2. Toss the cubed sweet potatoes in the salt, paprika, garlic, and avocado oil. Make sure that the potatoes are well-coated.

3. Lay the sweet potatoes out on the baking sheet and cook them for 25 minutes, or until they become soft.

4. As the potatoes cook, add the salt, lime juice, jalapeno, cilantro, cashews, and water to a high-speed blender and mix until smooth.

5. To make the salad, divide the salad greens into two plates and top with the cooked sweet potatoes. Top with the dressing and toss everything together.

Asparagus Salad with Lemon Dressing

Serves: 2

Salad –

Pepper, .25 tsp

Sea salt, .5 tsp

Crushed garlic, 3 cloves

Diced onion, .5 c.

Diced asparagus stalks, 24

Avocado oil, 1 tsp

Dressing –

Pepper

Sea salt, .25 tsp

Lemon juice, 2 tbsp

Water, .5 c.

Raw cashews, .5 c.

Assembling –

Mixed salad greens, 2 c.

1. For the asparagus, warm the oil in a massive frying pan and put in the pepper, salt, garlic, onion bulb, then the asparagus. Prepare for five until seven minutes, or till the onion has become soft.

2. To make the dressing, add half of the cooked asparagus mixture to a blender along with the pepper, salt, lemon

juice, water, and cashews. Blend up they are smooth and creamy.

3. To make your salad, divide the mixed greens between two plates and top with the rest of the cooked asparagus. Top with the dressing and enjoy.

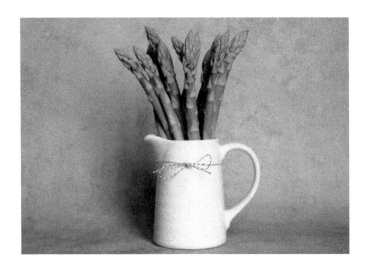

Dinner

Beefless Stew

Serves: 4

Dried oregano, 1 tsp

Diced celery, 2 stalks

Cubed large potato

Sliced carrot, 3 c.

Water, 2 c.

Vegetable broth, 3 c.

Pepper, one teaspoon

Seawater salt, one teaspoon

Mashed garlic, 2 bulbs

Diced onion, 1 c.

Avocado oil, 1 tbsp

Bay leaf

1. Heat up the avocado oil in an exceeding pot. Put in pepper, salt, garlic cloves, then onion bulbs. Cook everything for two to three minutes, or until the onion becomes soft.

2. Mix in the bay leaf, oregano, celery, potato, carrot, water, and broth. Allow this to come up to a simmer so that lower the heat down then prepare for 30-45 minutes, or until the carrots and potatoes become soft.

3. Taste and adjust the seasonings that you need to. If it is too thick, you can add some more water or broth.

4. Divide into four bowls and enjoy.

Emmenthal Soup

Serves: 2

Cayenne

Nutmeg

Pumpkin seeds, 1 tbsp

Chopped chives, 2 tbsp

Cubed Emmenthal cheese, 3 tbsp

Vegetable broth, 2 c.

Cubed potato, 1

Cauliflower pieces, 2 c.

1. Place the potato and cauliflower into a saucepan with the vegetable broth just until tender.

2. Place into a blender and puree.

3. Add in spices and adjust to taste.

4. Ladle into bowls, add in chives and cheese and stir well.

5. Garnish with pumpkin seeds. Enjoy.

Broccoli "Spaghetti"

Serves: 2

Pepper

Salt

Vegetable broth, 1 teaspoon

Oregano plant, 1 teaspoon

Juice - Lemon, 1 tablespoon

Sliced carrots, 3

Diced tomatoes, 3

Broccoli cut into floret, 1 head

Sliced pepper – red – bell, one

Sliced onion bulb, one

Diced garlic bulbs, two cloves

EVOO, 4 tbsp

Buckwheat pasta, 1 lb.

1. Place a pot of water on medium and add salt. Allow to boil and add in pasta. Prepare per box instructions. Empty out.

2. Place the broccoli into a different bowl and canopy with h2O. Prepare for five minutes.

3. Put a pan on normal heat and put in two tablespoons of olive oil into the skillet and warm. Put the bulbs, garlic, and onion then prepare till soft and scented. Remove from skillet then set to the side.

4. Add two more tablespoons of olive oil to the skillet and add carrots. Cook for five minutes, next put sweet pepper then prepare for another five minutes, now put in tomatoes then prepare for two minutes.

5. Completely drain the broccoli and add into the skillet with the rest of the vegetables. Put the onions and garlic back into the skillet.

6. Add vegetable broth, oregano, and lemon juice. Add some pepper and salt, taste and adjust seasonings if needed. Stir well to combine.

7. Place the cooked pasta onto a serving platter. Pour over vegetable mixture and toss to combine.

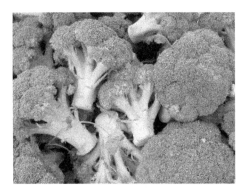

Indian Lentil Curry

Serves: 4 to 6

Lime juice

Chopped cilantro

Salt

EVOO, 1 tbsp

Diced tomatoes, 2

Sliced onion, 1

Minced garlic, 1 clove

Grated ginger, 1 inch

Turmeric, .5 tsp

Cumin seeds, .5 tsp

Chopped green chilies, 2

Fine red lentils, 1 c.

1. Place lentils into a bowl, cover with water and let sit for six hours.

2. After six hours, drain the lentils completely.

3. Place a basin on normal warmth. Put in the lentils then cover with fresh water. Allow to boil. Add in turmeric. Lower heat and simmer until lentils are cooked to your doneness.

4. Pull out from the pot then to a basin. Put these to side.

5. In another pan on medium, warm up olive oil. Add turmeric, cumin, ginger, and onions. Cook until onions are soft and ginger and fragrant.

6. Add chilies and tomatoes, and cook. Add salt and cook for five minutes.

7. Pour lentil into this mixture and bring back to a simmer. As shortly it begins to cook, remove it from the hot temperature. Squeeze in some lemon

8. Sprinkle with cilantro and serve with rice.

Vegetables with Wild Rice

Serves: 4

Salt

Basil

Cilantro

Juice of one lime

Chopped chili pepper, 1

Vegetable broth, .5 c.

Bean sprouts, 1 c.

Chopped carrots, 2 c.

Beans – green - diced, 1 c.

Broccoli, cleaved, 1 c.

Pak Choi, 1 c.

Wild rice, 1 c.

1. Place all the chopped vegetables into a pan and add vegetable broth.

2. Steam fry the vegetables until they are cooked through but still crunchy.

3. Using a mortar and pestle grind up the chili, basil, and cilantro until it forms a paste. Add in lime juice and mix well.

4. Place the rice onto a serving platter. Add the vegetables on top and drizzle with dressing.

Tangy Lentil Soup

Serves: 4

Salt

Turmeric, .25 tsp

Minced garlic, 3 cloves

Grated ginger, 1.5-inch piece

Chopped tomato, 1

Chopped Serrano Chile pepper, 1

Rinsed red lentils, 2 c.

Topping:

Coconut yogurt, .25 c.

1. Place the lentils in a colander and place under running water. Rinse until free from dirt and stones.

2. Pour rinsed lentils into a pot. Add enough water to cover lentils. Place the pot over medium heat and allow to boil.

3. Lower heat and simmer for ten minutes.

4. Put in the leftover contents then mix properly to blend.

5. Still, cook until lentils are soft.

6. Garnish with a spoonful of coconut yogurt.

Mushroom Leek Soup

Serves: 4

Sherry vinegar, 1.5 tbsp

Almond milk, .5 c.

Coconut cream, .66 c.

Vegetable broth, 3 c.

Chopped dill, 1 tbsp

Pepper

Salt

Almond flour, 5 tbsp

Cleaned, sliced mushrooms, 7 c.

Minced garlic, 3 cloves

Chopped leeks, 2.75 c.

Vegetable oil, 3 tbsp

1. Place a Dutch oven on medium and warm the oil. Add in the leeks together with garlic bulb then prepare till soft.

2. Put in the mushrooms, stir and cook an additional 10 minutes.

3. Add salt, dill, pepper, and flour. Stir well, until combined.

4. Put in soup and cause it to simmer. Lessen heat and put in rest of the ingredients. Stir well. Cook an additional ten minutes.

5. Serve warm with almond flour bread.

Fresh Veggie Pizza

Serves: 4

Crust –

Garlic bulb flavored powder, 0.5 teaspoon

Seawater salt, 0.5 teaspoon

Coconut oil, 3 tbsp

Almond flour, 1.25 c.

Tahini-Bee Spread –

Pepper, pinch

Sea salt, pinch

Garlic, 2 cloves

Juice - Lemon, one tablespoon

Avocado oil, one tablespoon

Middle eastern paste, one tablespoon

Peeled and cubed beets, 2

1. Start by placing your oven to 375. Place some parchment on a sheet tray.

2. Stir together the salt, garlic powder, coconut oil, and almond flour.

3. Place this on the sheet tray and squeeze into the shape of a ball. Place another piece of parchment on top and roll out the dough into 7x7 square. Bake for 14 minutes, or until it starts to brown.

4. As the crust bakes, add the pepper, salt, garlic, lemon juice, avocado oil, tahini, and beets to a food processor. Mix until it becomes creamy.

5. To make your pizza, spread the crust with beet sauces and then top with your favorite alkaline friendly veggies. Slice into four and enjoy.

Spicy Lentil Burgers

Serves: 4

Avocado oil, 1 tbsp

Coconut flour, 1 tbsp

Crushed garlic, 2 cloves

Diced jalapeno

Chopped cilantro, .5 c.

Diced onion, .5 c.

Pepper, .5 tsp

Sea salt, .5 tsp

Almond flour, .5 c.

Dry lentils, .5 c.

1. Cook the lentils following the directions on the package and set them to the side to cool off.

2. Mix together the garlic, jalapeno, cilantro, onion, pepper, salt, almond flour, and lentils until everything is well combined.

3. Add half of the lentil mixture to a food processor and process until it reaches a paste-like consistency.

4. Pour this back into the bowl with the rest of the lentil mixture and stir everything together. The mixture will be very moist. Stir in the coconut flour to help get rid of the moisture and to help them hold together.

5. Divide the mixture into fourths. Squeeze one-fourth of the mixture in your hands to flatten it out into a burger shape. Do this for the three remaining sections.

6. Warm up the oil in an exceedingly massive pot and put in the burgers. Prepare the burgers on 4 to 6 minutes on both sides, or until they have turned golden. When you flip them, do so carefully so that they don't fall apart. Enjoy.

Roasted Cauliflower Wraps

Serves: 2

Cauliflower –

Pepper, .25 tsp

Sea salt, .25 tsp

Garlic powder, .5 tsp

Nutritional yeast, .25 c.

Almond flour, .25 c.

Avocado oil, 1 tbsp

Bite-size cauliflower florets, 2 c.

Sauce –

Sea salt

Apple cider vinegar, 2 tbsp

Garlic, 2 cloves

Habanero pepper

Cubed mango, 1 c.

Assembling –

Collard greens, 2 leaves

Mixed salad greens, 1 c.

1. Start by placing your kitchen appliance to three hundred and fifty degrees then put a few papers on a cooking film.

2. To prepare your cauliflower, toss the cauliflower in the avocado oil and make sure they are evenly coated.

3. Into a container, combine along the all the seasonings: pepper, salt, garlic powder, healthy fungus, together with the almond flour.

4. Sprinkle the breading over the cauliflower and toss everything together making sure that the cauliflower is well-coated. Spread across the cooking film.

5. Cook it on about thirty up to thirty-five minutes, either that or till the cauliflower is soft.

6. As the cauliflower bakes, add the salt, vinegar, garlic, habanero, and mango to your blender and mix until well-combined. Make sure that you use some gloves or wash your hands really well when it comes to handling the habanero.

7. To assemble, divide the mixed salad greens between the collard leaves, top with the cauliflower and drizzle on the sauce. Wrap everything up like a burrito and enjoy.

Sliced Sweet Potato with Artichoke and Pepper Spread

Serves: 4

Pepper, .25 tsp

Salt, .5 tsp

Avocado oil, 6 tsp – divided

Quartered red bell pepper

Unpeeled sweet potatoes, 2 sliced into 4 lengthwise slices

Garlic, 2 cloves

Artichoke hearts, 14 oz can

1. Start by placing the oven to 350. Place some parchment on a sheet tray and set to the side.

2. Lay the bell pepper and sweet potato on the sheet tray and top them with two teaspoons of avocado oil, a pinch of pepper, and a pinch of salt.

3. Bake them for 30 minutes. Turn it over and cook to an additional fifteen minutes.

4. Add the roasted red bell pepper to a food processor along with the garlic, artichoke hearts, pepper, salt, and the remaining avocado oil. Pulse until combined but still a little chunky. Adjust any seasonings that you need.

5. Top the slices of sweet potato with the spread and enjoy.

Scallop Onion and Potato Bake

Serves: 4

Cashew Cheese Sauce –

Sea salt, .5 tsp

Nutritional yeast, .5 c.

Almond milk, 1 c.

Raw cashews, 1 c.

Scallop Bake –

Chopped tarragon, 1 tbsp

Pepper, 1 teaspoon

Seawater salt, one teaspoon

Oil – Avocado, one tablespoon

Chopped tiny onion bulbs, 1.5

Thinly sliced new potatoes, 8

1. To make the cheese sauce, add the cashews to a bowl and cover with room temperature water. Allow them to soak for 15 to 20 minutes and then drain and rinse.

2. Blend together the cashews with the remaining cheese sauce ingredients until smooth and creamy. Set to the side until later.

3. Start by heating the oven to 375.

4. Combine the onions and potatoes together in a bowl with the avocado oil. Toss in the tarragon, pepper, and salt, making sure everything is well coated.

5. Using an 8-inch square baking dish, place in the potato and onion mixture in the dish. Try your best to arrange them in nice rows. This doesn't have to be perfect.

6. Bake everything for 45 minutes, or until the potatoes become soft

7. Take it out of the oven and top with the cheese sauce. Divide between four plates and enjoy. You can also slide this, and cook inside the kitchen appliance on about 5 minutes in order to heat the caseous sauce through before serving.

Spicy Cilantro and Coconut Soup

Serves: 2

Cilantro leaves, 2 tbsp

Jalapeno

Lime juice, 1 tbsp

Full-fat coconut milk, 13.5 oz can

Sea salt, .25 tsp

Crushed garlic, 3 cloves

Diced onion, .5 c.

Avocado oil, 2 tbsp

1. Add the avocado oil to a medium pan and heat. Add in the salt, garlic, and onion, cooking for three to five minutes, either that or till the onion bulbs get to be smooth.

2. Put in the onion mixture, cilantro, jalapeno, lime juice, and coconut milk to a blender and mix until it becomes creamy.

3. Pour into a bowl and enjoy.

Tarragon Soup

Serves: 2

Chopped fresh tarragon, 2 tbsp

Celery stalk

Raw cashews, .5 c.

Lemon juice, 1 tbsp

Full-fat coconut milk, 13.5 oz can

Pepper, .5 tsp – divided

Sea salt, .5 tsp – divided

Crushed garlic, 3 cloves

Diced onion, .5 c.

Avocado oil, 1 tbsp

1. Add the oil to a medium pan and warm it up. Put in all the seasonings: pepper, salt, garlic bulbs, together with onion bulbs then prepare approximately three to five minutes, or until the onions turn soft.

2. Using a high-speed blender, add the onion mixture, tarragon, celery, cashews, lemon juice, and coconut milk. Blend everything together until smooth. Taste and adjust the seasonings as you need to.

3. Divide into two bowls and enjoy. You can also add back into a pot and heat through before serving.

Asparagus and Artichoke Soup

Serves: 4

Stemmed and halved artichoke hearts, 1 can

Almond milk, 2 c.

Pepper, .5 tsp

Sea salt, .5 - .75 tsp

Vegetable broth, 2 c.

Diced asparagus, 8 stalks

Cubed potatoes, 1 c.

Crushed garlic, 2 cloves

Avocado oil, 1 tbsp

Diced onion, .5 c.

1. Add the garlic, avocado oil, and onion in a skillet and cook for a few minutes, either that or till the onion bulbs have smoothened and weakened.

2. Put in the cooked veggies to a pot and add in the pepper, salt, vegetable broth, asparagus, and potatoes. Stir everything together and let it come up to a simmer. Lower the hot temperature and boil gently on about eighteen up to twenty minutes, either that or till the potatoes have become soft. Add in some extra broth if you find that you need to so that the liquid stays about an inch over the veggies.

3. Set the pot away from the fire then let it chill.

4. Using a blender, mix up the cooled soup with the artichokes and almond milk until everything is well-combined and smooth. Adjust any of the seasonings that you need to. You can add extra broth or milk to thick it out if needed.

5. Pour back into the pot and let it warm over low until ready to serve.

Mint and Berry Soup

Serves: 1

Sweetener –

Water, .25 c – plus more if needed

Unrefined whole cane sugar, .25 c.

Soup –

Water, .5 c.

Mixed berries, 1 c.

Mint leaves, 8

Lemon juice, 1 tsp

1. Add the water and sugar to a small pot and cook, stirring constantly, until the sugar has dissolved. Allow this to cool.

2. Add the mint leaves, lemon juice, water, berries, and the cooled sugar mixture to a blender. Mix everything together until smooth.

3. Pour into a basin then put in the refrigerator till the broth is completely chilled. This will take about 20 minutes.

4. Enjoy.

Mushroom Soup

Serves: 2

Full-fat coconut milk, 13.5 oz can

Vegetable broth, 1 c.

Pepper, .5 tsp

Sea salt, .75 tsp

Crush garlic clove

Diced onion, 1 cup

Cut up cremini mushrooms, 1 cup

Cut up Chinese black mushrooms, one cup

Avocado oil, 1 tbsp

Coconut aminos, 1 tbsp

Dried thyme, .5 tsp

1. Warm up the grease in a very massive pan then put in all the seasonings: pepper, salt, garlic, onion bulb, and mushrooms. Boil and prepare everything along for a few minutes, either that or till the onions turn soft.

2. Mix in the coconut aminos, thyme, coconut milk, and vegetable broth. Lower the fire down then allow the broth to boil on approximately a quarter-hour. Mix the broth from time to time.

3. Taste and adjust any of the seasonings that you need to. Divide into two bowls and enjoy.

Potato Lentil Stew

Serves: 4

Chopped oregano sprigs, 2 sprigs

Diced celery stalk

Cubed and peeled potato, 1 c.

Sliced carrots, 2

Dry lentils, 1 c.

Spicy condiment / Pepper, one teaspoon

Seawater salt, one to 1.5 teaspoon

Mashed garlic bulbs, two buds

Diced onion, .5 c.

Avocado oil, 2 tbsp

Full-fat coconut milk, 13.5 oz can

Vegetable broth, 5 c – divided

Chopped tarragon, 2 sprigs

1. Using a big cooking utensil, warm the avocado grease together with putting in seasonings: pepper, salt, garlic bulbs, together with onion. Cook for three to five minutes, or until the onion has become soft.

2. Mix in the tarragon, oregano, celery, potato, carrots, lentils, and 2 ½ cups of the vegetable broth. Mix everything together.

3. Enable the casserole to return up to heat and then lower the fire down. Let this cook, stirring often. Add in extra

vegetable broth in half cup portions as needed to make sure that the lentils have enough liquid to cook. Let the stew cook for 20 to 25 minutes, or until the lentils and potatoes are soft.

4. Set the stew off the heat and mix in the coconut milk. Divide into four bowls and enjoy.

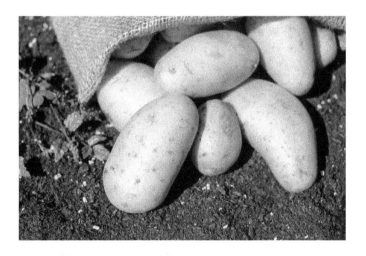

Snacks

Thanksgiving Pudding

Serves: 8

Coconut whipped cream

Cored, diced apples, .5 c.

Raisins, .5 c.

Salt

Cinnamon, 1 tsp

Unsweetened coconut milk, .5 c.

Unsweetened pumpkin puree, 1 can

1. You need to warm your oven to 350.

2. Place the nutmeg, salt, coconut milk, cinnamon, and pumpkin into kitchen appliance then pat till soft and even.

3. Put in the apples and raisins. Pulse a few times to combine.

4. Pour mixture into a 9-inch pie plate.

5. Place into the oven for one hour until the top is cracked just slightly.

6. Serve topped with whipped coconut cream.

Banana Muffins

Serves: 12

Split and deseeded vanilla bean, 1

Salt

Baking soda, 2 tsp

Melted coconut oil, .25 c.

Coconut flour, .5 c.

Creamy almond butter, .5 c.

Dates, 1 c.

Ripe bananas, 2.

Cooking spray

1. You need to warm your oven to 350. Place paper liners into a cupcake tin.

2. Place the dates and bananas into a food processor and process until well-blended. Add in vanilla bean seed, hydrogen carbonate, salt, coconut flour, copra oil, then almond butter. Process until batter forms.

3. Place batter into muffin tin until it is about 75 percent full.

4. Place into oven and bake eighteen minutes. The small cakes are finished once toothpick is placed in the center and turns out neat. Allow to cool slightly and enjoy.

Almost Crispy Rice Treatlets

Serves: 12

Brown rice cereal, 4 c.

Salt

Split and scraped vanilla bean, 1

Coconut oil, .25 c.

Brown rice syrup, .66 c.

Cooking spray

1. Using a nine-inch cooking platter, sprinkle it with some spray for cooking.

2. Put the saucepan on medium. Add in coconut oil and rice syrup and allow to boil for one minute.

3. Add salt and vanilla bean seed.

4. Place the rice cereal into a bowl. Pour syrup mixture over. Mix well until all cereal is coated.

5. Run through the readied pan. Put cooking spray into your hands then push the blended concoction to the pan to make an even layer.

6. Allow to sit for 45 minutes.

Fruit Crumble

Serves: 6

Salt

Softened coconut oil, one tablespoon

No-sugar grated coconut, .5 c.

Raw almonds, 1.5 c.

Split and scraped vanilla bean, 1

Stevia, 1 packet

Chopped summer fruits of choice like strawberries, plums, blueberries, etc., 2 c.

Cooking spray

1. You need to warm your oven to 350. Spray a nine-inch baking dish and set to the side.

2. Put a saucepan on medium heat. Add stevia, vanilla bean, and fruits. Stir well and allow to boil.

3. Add the coconut oil, salt, and almonds to a food processor. Pulse until crumbly mixture forms.

4. Place the fruit into a baking dish.

5. Top with almond mixture. Place in the oven for 15 minutes.

Pumpkin Crackers

Serves: 6

Alkaline water, 1.33 c.

Melted coconut oil, 3 tbsp

Salt

Psyllium husk powder, 1 tbsp

Sesame seeds, .33 c.

Flaxseed, .75 c.

Sunflower seeds, .75 c.

Pumpkin pie spice, 2 tbsp

Coconut flour, .33 c.

1. You need to warm your oven to 300. Take a cookie sheet and line it with paper.

2. Place every dry ingredient to a basin then stir well to combine.

3. Add in oil and water, and mix well. Allow the flour mixture to rest for 3 minutes.

4. Lay the flour mixture out onto prepared cookie sheet.

5. Place into the oven for 30 minutes. Lower temperature to 225 and continue to bake another 30 minutes.

6. Take out of the oven and crack the bread into pieces.

Apple Crisps

Serves: 4

Cinnamon, .5 tsp

White sugar, 1.5 tsp

Cored, thinly sliced apples, 2

1. You need to warm your kitchen appliance to two hundred twenty-five degrees. Lay out a cooking film with paper.

2. Combine cinnamon spice together with sugar together in a bowl.

3. Put apple slices into sugar mixture and toss to evenly coat.

4. Spread coated apples onto a prepared baking sheet. Place in oven for 45 minutes.

5. Take out of the oven and allow to cool slightly.

Peanut Butter Bars

Serves: 6

Vanilla, .5 tsp

Peanut butter, .5 c.

Swerve Sweetener, .25 c.

Almond butter, 2 oz

Almond flour, .75 c

1. Place all ingredients into a bowl and mix well until well-combined.

2. Place into a six-inch square pan. Press down firmly.

3. Place in the refrigerator for 30 minutes.

4. Take out of the refrigerator, evenly slice and serve.

Zucchini Chips

Serves: 4

Thinly sliced zucchini, 2

Pepper – red - gratings, three tablespoons

Pepper - regular

Onion flavored powder, one teaspoon

Garlic flavored powder, one teaspoon

Oil - vegetable, 1.66 cup

1. You need to warm your oven to 350.

2. Place the spices and oil into a bowl and mix well. Add in the zucchini and toss to evenly coat.

3. Place into a zip top bag and seal. Place in the refrigerator for ten minutes.

4. Take out of the refrigerator and spread sliced zucchini onto a greased baking sheet.

5. Place in the oven and bake 15 minutes.

6. Carefully remove from oven and let cool slightly.

Cashew Cream Stuffed Mushrooms

Serves: 6

Mushrooms –

Pinch pepper

Pinch sea salt

Avocado oil, 1.5 tsp

Stemmed cremini mushrooms, 12

Stuffing –

Sea salt, .25 teaspoon

Apple vinegar, one teaspoon

Juice - Lemon, 0.25 cup

Garlic bulbs, two cloves

Raw cashews, 1 c.

1. To prepare the mushrooms, rinse and dry the mushroom caps.

2. Add the oil to a medium-size pan. Place in the mushroom caps and sprinkle on some pepper and salt. Sauté them for a couple of minutes, or until soft. Get rid of the liquid that has accumulated in the pan.

3. For the stuffing, add the salt, vinegar, lemon juice, garlic, and cashews in a blender and mix until it creates a thick paste.

4. Spoon this into the mushroom caps and enjoy.

Garlic Breadsticks

Serves: 12

Breadsticks –

Pepper, 0.5 teaspoon

Seawater salt, 0.5 teaspoon

Oregano, chopped, one tablespoon

Oil - avocado, one tablespoon

Almond flour, 2 c.

Ground flaxseed, 1 tbsp

Water, 3 tbsp

Topping –

Avocado oil, 1 tbsp

Pepper

Sea salt

Chopped fresh oregano, 1 tbsp

Crushed garlic, 4 cloves

1. Start by placing your oven to 350. Place some parchment on a sheet tray.

2. To fix the breadstick, whisk the water and flaxseed together to make the flax egg.

3. Stir together the pepper, salt, oregano, avocado oil, almond flour, and flax egg until they come together and forms a dough.

4. Place the mixture on your prepared sheet tray and form it into a ball. Set an additional piece of paper above then utilize a kitchen utensil to flat the dough out into a 5x8 inch rectangle.

5. To make the topping, mix together the pepper, salt, oregano, garlic, avocado oil together. Pour the garlic oil over the dough and spread it out with the rear of a spoon.

6. Cook the breadsticks to about eighteen up to twenty minutes, either that or till it starts to brown.

7. Remove and slice into 12 pieces. Enjoy.

Tarragon Crackers

Serves: 5

Garlic powder, .25 tsp

Pepper, 0.5 teaspoon

Seawater salt, 0.5 teaspoon

Oil – avocado, one tablespoon

Daisy plant herb, one tablespoon

Almond flour, 2 c.

Ground flaxseed, 1 tablespoon

Water, 3 tbsp

1. Start by heating your kitchen appliance to three hundred and fifty degrees. Put some paper on a cooking film tray.

2. Beat the water and flaxseed together to make your flax egg.

3. Stir the garlic powder, pepper, salt, avocado oil, tarragon, and almond flour into the flax egg. Make sure everything comes together.

4. Place this on the baking sheet and then form it into a ball with your hands. Lay another sheet of parchment on top and roll the dough out to a quarter inch thickness.

5. With a knife or pizza cutter, slice the dough into 60 squares.

6. Bake them for 12 to 14 minutes. They should golden on top. Turn them over then cook them for an additional 2 minutes.

7. Cool the crackers and then enjoy.

Pear Nachos with Almond Butter

Serves: 1

Unsweetened shredded coconut flakes, 1 to 2 tsp

Hemp seeds, 1 to 2 tsp

Water, 1 to 2 tbsp – if needed

Cinnamon, pinch

Vanilla bean powder, pinch

Unrefined whole cane sugar, 2 to 3 tsp

Almond butter, 2 tbsp

Sliced and unpeeled pear

Slivered almonds, 1 tbsp

1. Lay the pear slices on a plate.

2. To fix the drizzle, add the cinnamon, vanilla bean powder, sugar, and almond butter to a bowl and mix together until everything is well-combined. Depending on how thick your almond butter is, you may need to add some water to help thin it out. You only want it to be thin enough so that you can drizzle it.

3. Drizzle the almond butter over the sliced pears. Top with some almonds, coconut flakes, and hemp seeds and enjoy. You can also dip the pear slices in any extra drizzle that you may have.

Chewy Seed and Nut Bars

Serves: 16

Vanilla bean powder, 1 tsp

Brown rice syrup, .25 c.

Unrefined whole cane sugar, .5 c.

Hemp seeds, .5 c.

Sesame seeds, .5 c.

Raw pumpkin seeds, .5 c.

Raw almonds, .75 c.

Raw cashews, .75 c.

Pinch sea salt

Cinnamon, 1 tsp

1. Start by placing your oven to 350 and lay some parchment into an 8-inch baking pan.

2. Mix together the hemp seeds, sesame seeds, pumpkin seeds, almonds, and cashews together.

3. Add the salt, cinnamon, vanilla bean powder, brown rice syrup, and sugar to a small pot and heat. Cook and stir until the sugar dissolves.

4. Quickly pour this over the seeds and nuts, and mix together until everything is well-coated.

5. Pour into the prepared pan and flatten out into an even layer using your hands. Bake for 18 to 20 minutes.

6. Allow this to cool completely for 30 to 45 minutes. Cut into 16 squares.

Cinnamon Cashews

Serves: 4

Raw cashews, 1.5 c.

Vanilla bean powder, .25 tsp

Cinnamon, .25 tsp

Unrefined whole cane sugar, .5 c.

Water, .5 c

1. Place some parchment on a sheet tray and set to the side.

2. Add the vanilla bean powder, cinnamon, sugar, and water in a small pot and cook until the sugar dissolves.

3. Add in the cashews and turn the heat up to med-high. Cook, stirring constantly, for four to six minutes. Do not step away from this. The sugary liquid is going to thicken and stick to the cashews. If you step away, it could end up hardening incorrectly.

4. Once the liquid has cooked away, set this off the heat and spread out on the sheet tray. You can move the cashews so that none of them are touching or you can let them form little clusters.

5. Let them cool and enjoy.

Coconut and Vanilla Truffles

Serves: 12

Sea salt

Vanilla bean fine grains, two teaspoons

Cashew nut butter, two tablespoons

Coconut flour, two tablespoons

Brown rice syrup, .25 c.

Coconut oil, .25 c.

Unsweetened coconut flakes, 2 c.

1. Add the vanilla bean powder, cashew butter, coconut flour, brown rice syrup, coconut oil, coconut flakes, and salt to a food processor and pulse until it creates a sticky mixture.

2. Let the mixture sit in the refrigerator for around 15 minutes, or until it has firmed up so that it will hold the shape of a ball.

3. Roll tablespoonfuls into balls and place in a lidded container. Keep them in the refrigerator until you want to serve them. They will end up becoming soft if you leave them at room temperature.

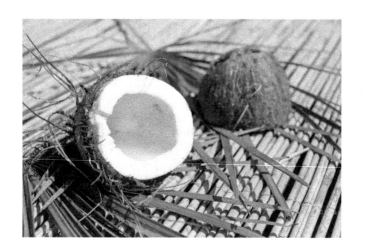

Cashew Butter Fudge

Serves: 16

Sesame seeds, hemp seeds, chia seeds, unsweetened shredded coconut flakes – optional toppings

Brown rice syrup, 2 tbsp

Melted coconut oil, .25 c.

Cashew butter, 1 c.

1. Stir the brown rice syrup, coconut oil, and cashew butter together until everything is well mixed.

2. Divide the fudge mixture between 16 mini muffin cups, filling them to about ¾ of the way full.

3. If you want, you can now top them with some sesame seeds, hemp seeds, chia seeds, or shredded coconut.

4. Place them in the freezer for a couple of hours to allow them to firm.

5. Keep them stored in the freezer until you want to enjoy one. They will become soft if they sit at room temperature.

Lime and Chia Seed Cookies

Serves: 12

Pinch sea salt

Brown rice syrup, .25 c.

Coconut flour, 2 tbsp

Chia seeds, two tablespoons

Juice - Lime, two tablespoons

Coconut oil, three up to four tablespoons – divided

Raw cashews, 2 c.

1. Start by placing your oven to 350 and place some parchment on a sheet pan.

2. Add two tablespoons of coconut oil and the cashews in a food processor and combine until you make cashew butter. This will take upwards of ten minutes and will go through several different steps. Stop every couple of minutes to scrape the sides down so that everything is blended evenly. You can add in more coconut oil if you need to, a tablespoon at a time, to make it creamier. Don't exceed four tablespoons.

3. Add the cashew butter to a bowl and add in the salt, brown rice syrup, coconut flour, chia seeds, and lime juice. Stir everything together.

4. Roll tablespoonfuls of the dough into balls and press them slightly into a disk shape. Place them on the sheet pan. Continue with the rest of the dough.

5. Bake the cookies for 12 minutes, making sure that they don't over-bake.

6. Let the cookies cool completely before taking them off the pan. They are going to be soft and crumbly when they first come out of the oven but will firm up as they cool. Enjoy.

Apple Crumble

Serves: 6

Apple Filling –

Juice from ¼ of a lemon

Cinnamon, .5 tsp

Brown rice syrup, 1 tbsp

Diced apple

Crumble –

Unrefined whole cane sugar, .5 c.

Almond flour, 2 c.

Ground flaxseed, 1 tbsp

Water, 3 tbsp

Pinch sea salt

Vanilla bean powder, pinch

Cinnamon, .5 tsp

Avocado oil, 1 tbsp

1. Start by setting your oven to 350. Place some parchment into a 9x5 inch loaf pan.

2. To prepare the apple filling, mix together the lemon juice, cinnamon, brown rice syrup, and apple and set to the side.

3. For the crumble, stir the water and flaxseed together to make the flax egg.

4. Mix together the salt, vanilla bean powder, cinnamon, avocado oil, sugar, almond flour, and flax egg till nicely blended.

5. Push down ½ of the crushed combination underneath the loaf pan.

6. Top the crumble with the apple filling and spread out evenly. Sprinkle the rest of the crumble over top of the apples.

7. Bake this for 20 to 25 minutes and enjoy.

Pumpkin Seed Cookies

Serves: 20

Sea salt, .25 tsp

Baking soda, .5 tsp

Brown rice syrup, 2 tbsp

Raw pumpkin seeds, .5 c.

Almond flour, .5 c.

Coconut oil, .5 c.

Raw cashews, 2 c.

1. Start by placing your oven to 350 and place some parchment on a sheet pan.

2. Add the coconut oil and cashews in the food processor and mix until the cashews turn into cashew butter. This is going to take around ten minutes and will go through several different phases. Stop every few minutes to scrape the bowl down so that everything processes completely. This will make around a cup of cashew butter.

3. Add the cashew butter to a bowl and stir in the salt, baking soda, brown rice syrup, pumpkin seeds, and almond flour.

4. Roll tablespoonfuls of the dough into balls and press them slightly to flatten. Lay them on the sheet pan and continue with the rest of the cookie dough.

5. Bake the cookies for 10 to 12 minutes, making sure that they don't burn.

6. Let the cookies cool completely before taking them off of the sheet pan. They are going to be soft and crumbly when they first come out but they will firm up as they cool.

7. Keep them in a lidded container and in the fridge so that the coconut oil doesn't melt.

Juices

The Green Machine

Serves: 1

Green apple, .5

Peeled lemon, .5

Small bunch parsley

Celery stalk

Cucumber

Dandelion greens, 2 c.

1. Juice everything and enjoy.

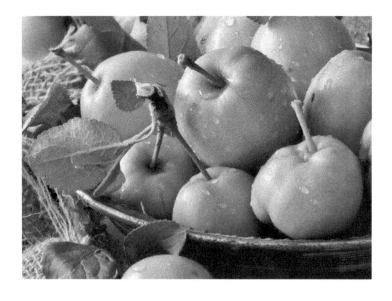

Ginger Spinach Juice

Serves: 1

Pinch sea salt

Knob of ginger

Cored green apple, .5

Peeled lemon

Scrubbed carrot

Celery stalk

English cucumber, .5

Handful baby spinach

1. Juice all of the ingredients together, stir and enjoy.

Green Juice

Serves: 1

Handful dill

Handful mint

Chunk ginger

Lime, .5

Romaine, 3 leaves

Zucchini

Celery stalk

Large cucumbers, 2

1. Juice all of the ingredients together, stir and enjoy.

Morning Energy Juice

Serves: 2

Half an apple

Red bell pepper

Ginger, .5 inch

Carrots, 2

Baby spinach, 2 c.

Melted coconut oil, 1 tbsp

Juice of a lemon

Garlic clove

Half fennel

1. Chop and wash the pepper, fennel, carrots, and greens.

2. Juice them together and then pour into a large container. Mix in the coconut oil and lemon juice. Mix and divide into two glasses.

Full Energy Juice

Serves: 2

Olive oil, 2 tbsp

Chili powder and curry powder to taste

Black pepper

Salt

Large avocado

Tomatoes, 2

Zucchini, 2

Garlic cloves, 2

Carrots, 2

Kale, 2 c.

1. Chop and wash the tomatoes, zucchini, carrots, and kale. Juice them and then juice the garlic.

2. Chop the avocado and blend the juice and avocado together in a blender and then mix in the spices.

Anti-Inflammatory Juice

Serves: 1

Red bell peppers, 2

Apple

Beets, 2

Nutmeg, .5 tsp

Cinnamon, .5 tsp

Chia seeds, two tablespoons

Oil - coconut, two tablespoons

Milk - coconut, one cup

Ginger spice, one inch

Greens of choice, 2 c.

1. Chop and wash the veggies and then juice them along
   with the ginger. Stir in the coconut milk, nutmeg, and
   cinnamon. Sprinkle with the chia seeds and enjoy.

Green Tea

Serves: 1

Juice of a lemon

Juice of 2 grapefruits

Green tea, 1 c.

1. Stir all of the ingredients together. You can add some stevia to sweeten if you would like.

Party Juice

Serves: 2

Juice of a lemon

Pear

Ginger, 1 inch

Half fennel

Broccoli florets, a few

Kale, .5 c.

Peeled cucumbers, 4

1. Clean and chop your veggies and peel the ginger and cucumber. Juice everything together and stir in the lemon juice. Divide into two glasses and enjoy.

Fat Burn Juice

Serves: 2

Cinnamon, .5 tsp

Cucumber

Beets, 2

Kale, 1 c.

Baby spinach, 1 c.

Alkaline water – if needed

1. Clean and chop your veggies and juice them together. Mix in the cinnamon. If you find that the taste is too intense, you can mix in some water to dilute it slightly. Divide into two glasses and enjoy.

Healthy Kidneys

Serves: 1

Coconut water, .5 c.

Cucumber

Kale, 1 c.

Red bell pepper

Ginger root, .5 inch

Turmeric root, .5 inch

1. Clean and chop up the ingredients and juice them together. Stir in the coconut water and enjoy.

Liver Lover

Serves: 2

Pinch salt

Ginger, 1 inch

Garlic clove

Pressed flax oil, 2 tbsp

Alkaline water, .5 c.

Parsley, .5 c.

Juice of 2 lemons

Juice of 2 grapefruits

1. Blend everything together and stir in the salt and oil. Divide into two glasses and enjoy.

Mind and Body Juice

Serves: 1

Olive oil, 1 tbsp

Fennel, .5

Turmeric, .5 inch

Ginger, .5 inch

Broccoli florets, a few

Cucumbers, 2

Celery, 2 stalks

Swiss chard, .5 c.

Kale, .5 c.

1. Wash all of the veggies and chop. Juice everything together and stir in the oil. Drink and enjoy.

Maca Juice

Serves: 2

Olive oil, 1 tbsp

Maca powder, .5 tsp

Juice of a lemon

Parsley, .5 c.

Ginger, .5 inch

Fennel slices

Tomatoes, 3

Watercress, .5 c.

1. Clean and chop your veggies and then juice them together. Put to a crystal ware then blend in with the lemon juice, oil, then maca powder. Divide into two glasses and enjoy.

Metabolism Booster

Serves: 1

Chia seeds, 1 tbsp

Mint leaves, .25 c.

Ginger, .5 inch

Cinnamon, .5 tsp

Beet

Celery, 2 stalks

Small carrot

Juice of a grapefruit

Spinach, 1 c.

1. Clean all of the ingredients and chop the carrot, spinach, beet, and celery. Juice everything together. Stir in the grapefruit juice and top with the chia seeds.

Purple Juice

Serves: 1

Pinch salt

Olive oil, 1 tsp

Juice of a lime

Juice of a lemon

Beet

Mint, .25 c.

Parsley, .25 c.

Medium cucumbers, 2

Celery, 2 stalks

1. Clean and chop the ingredients. Juice everything together and then stir in the salt, oil, lime, and lemon juice. Enjoy.

Smoothies

Kale and Avocado Smoothie

Serves: 2

Hemp seeds, 1 tbsp

Roughly chopped banana, .5

Roughly chopped avocado, .5

Stemmed kale stalks, 2

Almond milk, 1.5 c.

1. Simply place the ingredients to your blender and mix until smooth. Divide the smoothie into two glasses and enjoy.

Triple Berry Protein

Serves: 1

Pumpkin protein powder, 3 tsp

Blackberries, .33 c.

Blueberries, .33 c.

Raspberries, .33 c.

Coconut milk, 1.5 c.

1. Simply put each of the contents of the smoothie to your liquidizer then blend along till soft and nicely blended.

Pina Colada Smoothie

Serves: 1

Ice cubes, 1 c.

Pineapple chunks, 2.5 c.

Unsweetened coconut milk, .5 c.

1. Add the pineapple, coconut milk, and ice into the blender. Process until smooth and creamy.

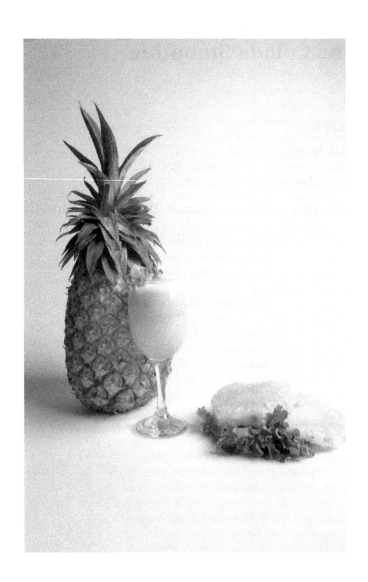

Raspberry Papaya Mango Smoothie

Serves: 1

Chopped, seeded papaya, .5

Frozen mango, .75 c.

Raspberries, .25 c.

1. Put everything to the liquidizer then process till even and creamy.

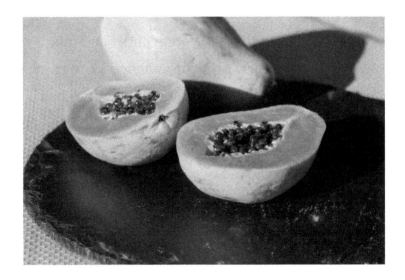

Cherry and Watermelon Smoothie

Serves: 2

Ice cubes, 5-7

Lime juice, one tablespoon

Brown rice sweetening, one tablespoon

Coconut milk, 1 c.

Dark sweet cherries, 10

Cubed watermelon, 2 c.

1. Simply add everything to your blender and mix everything together, using just enough ice to reach your desired consistency. Once smooth, pour into two glasses and enjoy.

Kiwi Hemp Seed Smoothie

Serves: 1

Ice cubes, 5-7

Hemp seeds, 2 tbsp

Blueberries, 1 c fresh or frozen

Peeled and chopped kiwi

Almond milk, 1.5 c.

1. Simply blend all of the ingredients together with enough ice to reach your desired consistency. Once everything is well combined, pour into a glass and enjoy.

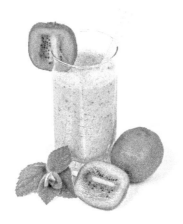

Mango Smoothie

Serves: 2

Ice cubes, 5-7

Raw cashews, .25 c.

Peeled and chopped kiwi

Chopped mango, .5 c.

Coconut milk, 1.5 c.

1. You will need a high-speed blender for this smoothie to help break up the cashews. Simply blend all of the ingredients together with enough ice to reach your desired consistency. Once well combined and smooth, pour into two glasses and serve.

Kick Start Your Diet

Starting the alkaline diet is a lot easier said than done. This section gives you ideas on how to make this new lifestyle easy to begin and stick with. Try to remember these simple principles:

- Take it slow, take baby steps, take it day by day instead of going full throttle the first day.

- Nobody is perfect. You need to enjoy life. Take a day off, enjoy your favorite treats and foods and get out there and socialize.

- You don't have to change your personality to be healthy.

This alkaline lifestyle is meant to fit into your life, not the other way around.

Five Simple Steps

- Hydration

Research shows that 90 percent of people are dehydrated and don't even know it. This has the possibility of creating a big influence on your standard of living. Many people don't like to drink water and this is probably the reason they don't feel well most of the time.

Being hydrated makes a huge difference to your immunity, vitality, energy, and health. Everything gets influenced by the quality and quantity of the water they drink. Try to filter your water until it has a pH between 8 and 9.5.

Steps to keep you hydrated:

1. Drink herbal teas like nettle and peppermint.

2. Drink lemon water: Take two cups of filtered, lukewarm water, and juice from one-fourth of a lemon. This will help cleanse your digestive system, buffer excess acids, and ignite your metabolism. As we learned before lemons are acidic in their natural state but once it gets into your system it becomes alkaline.

3. Try to drink between 6 and 18 cups of water daily. Consider your weight then split it in ½. With this range, consume those several ounces of water every day.

- Eat Green

The alkaline is all about alkaline foods. There is some conflicting information about what foods are alkaline and acid. If you stick to the lists that were given above and the 80/20 rule, you shouldn't have any problems figuring out what you should and shouldn't eat.

- Transition

Go slowly. Just about everybody out there who tries a new diet will go 100 percent out from day one but will fail within one week and it usually only takes one day.

This alkaline lifestyle isn't restrictive, isn't difficult, and is fairly simple when you have gotten your body used to it. If you try to be perfect from the beginning, you won't be able to experiment, learn, and figure out meals that work for you and your family. You might end up feeling restricted, fed up, and hungry.

It is better to transition slowly by sticking with it for a long time instead of being perfect for a couple of days and then crashing.

- Oxygen

If you can learn to do simple breathing exercises a couple times each day, you are giving your body a big hand in removing excess acids from your body. It also lets you relax, visualize, focus your mind, and just stop for the moment. Just find a place where you can sit comfortably, close your eyes, and follow this breathing exercise:

1. Inhale like this: 1, 2 (every two counts)

2. Hold onto your air for 8 counts.

3. Exhale for 4 counts.

4. Go through this exercise ten times.

- Supplements

This is the part of the alkaline diet that confuses most people. There are many supplements out there, and they all promise various things. Each one claims it is better than the next one. Here are some supplements that are recommended:

1. Omega Oils

Taking an omega-3 supplement or an oil blend that includes omega-9, 6, and 3 would be very beneficial.

2. Alkaline minerals

The best way our bodies can buffer acids is by alkaline minerals like calcium, potassium, magnesium, and sodium.

3. Alkaline water

You can create alkaline water in several different ways: adding lemon juice to your water, using pH drops, or a water ionizer.

4. Green powder

This is a combination of sprouts, vegetables, fruits, and powdered grasses while focusing on barley grass and wheat grass.

This diet is simple if you take it slow. Aim for 80/20 instead of trying to be perfect. If you allow yourself to have fun and have treats, it will make the transition smoother. Enjoy your life, have fun, and take it easy.

Keep things simple and if you make a mistake, don't beat yourself up. Take a walk, get focused, and start over. You have the rest of your life so make it interesting. Enjoy it with vitality, energy, and health that this new alkaline lifestyle will bring.

Living the Alkaline Life

Your significant other offers you a bowl of their fettuccine Alfredo. Your friend hands you a plate with a huge slice of apple pie with a scoop of ice cream on top. Your boss sends you to a conference out of town. It is hard to stick with a healthy eating plan with the people around you aren't eating healthy or if you find yourself in a situation where you might not have control of what you eat. Don't let this stress you out. Here are some tips that can help you remain on track without making others feel bad and will help you get around other food situations that might be a bit challenging.

- Happy hour

Alcoholic drinks are calorie bombs and are very acidic on the body. You need to know your options and make wise choices. If you need something bubbly, pick seltzer water which is just water with bubbles added. What's more is it is zero calories. Tonic water has 120 calories that come from nothing but sugar. When your friends want to go out, be the designated driver, your friends will thank you and won't question your choices.

- Work celebrations

Having food in the workplace is inevitable. Instead of stressing about it or letting it derail you, figure out in advance how you are going to deal with any temptations that might pop up. The best strategy is to find a support group of coworkers who are also trying to eat clean. With everyone together, you can all politely decline or bring healthier alternatives like a vegetable and fruit platter. Keep healthy snacks at your desk or in the office refrigerator so you will have something healthy when other people try to indulge. Some examples are sliced vegetables, hummus, vegetable soups, apples, whole almonds, almond butter to dip celery sticks in, and kale chips.

- Dealing with hunger

Letting yourself get hungry is the fastest way to get off track with the alkaline lifestyle. Establish an eating plan with snacks and meals. Some people need their snacks and some like to snack after every meal. You should allow natural hunger to be your guide, stress can sometimes override your natural cues but they lead us to ignore the need for nourishment. Take one day every week to get your snacks and meals planned out. This will keep your body fueled all day.

- Business dinners or lunches

You have to make your own choices and it doesn't matter what your coworkers are doing. You have free will to choose what you want to drink and eat. Every restaurant will have salads and vegetables on their menu. Many are willing to accommodate special diets. If they have a vegetable soup on the menu, order that plus add a salad or vegetables to make protein the side dish instead of the main meal. Most people don't like to appear as "high maintenance" where they work. You can make healthy boundaries for yourself and have control over what you eat. Remember the 80/20 rule if your choices aren't as ideal as they could be.

- Weekends

Having structured routines for the week helps you stick to an eating plan. When weekends roll around it can throw a wrench into the plans. There is room for splurges but remember your health goals when making choices. Stay consistent and focused. Try to continue with exercising and regular meals. You can splurge every now and then but remember portion sizes. Begin each day with a healthy breakfast, stick to the basics, and keep things simple like including vegetables, fruits, healthy fats, and lean proteins that will help you feel fuller for longer.

- Traveling

When you are away from home, sticking to a diet can be hard. You can do it if you are proactive. Take some time to research supermarkets and restaurants before you go. Pack some healthy snacks that won't spoil like apples and almonds. If you are traveling in a car, pack a cooler with tubers, avocados, seeds, fruits, and vegetables. If you will be staying at a hotel, call and request a microwave and refrigerator if they don't come with the room. You can stick to your alkaline lifestyle; all you need to do is commit, plan, and research.

- Sabotage

If your significant other doesn't approve of your new lifestyle, they might feel threatened and this causes a negative reaction. To stop this from happening, ask for their support before you begin the alkaline diet. Let them know you are living a healthier life and would like to have their support. Tell them that helping you prepare healthy meals is a great way for them to show their love. Ask them to help you find recipes and let them help plan the menu.

- Holidays

Holidays are rough on our waistlines even if you are trying to follow a special eating plan. The best thing to do is be proactive and prepare dishes that are alkaline-friendly to share at your gatherings. Remember, it is okay to eat some treats, just remember portion sizes and fill your plate with more vegetables and healthier foods.

A Few More Tips

By this point, you should have a good idea of what an alkaline diet is and how to get started. As with any diet, though, it can be difficult to really get into it and not allow yourself to fall back into old habits. To make sure you kick start your diet the best way possible, here are just a few more tips that can help to make the transition a little easier.

1. Fall in love with healthy foods

Instead of getting rid of all the foods that you love right off the bat, start to slowly add in healthy foods that will help to boost your energy and mood, like kiwi, grapefruit, berries, and green veggies. Place a chart on your fridge that shows you ten servings of good foods. Each time you eat one of the healthy foods, write it down. This will help to lower your cravings for refined sweets.

2. Fight off your cravings with healthy snacks

When you experience a craving, eat some fiber or something that is sour. This lowers your glycemic index and controls your craving. Try to keep healthy snacks on head like fruits to stay away from acidic foods like sugar and flour.

3. Start off your day with a meal that is heavy in protein to fight off sugar cravings

Instead of making dinner your biggest meal of the day, make breakfast your biggest meal. People in Japan are historically healthy, and they begin their day with fish and veggies. If you like carbs, have them first thing during the day or right have you workout. Doing this will help to keep your full and alert until your next meal without experiencing cravings. In order to figure out what your daily protein needs are, take you weight in kilograms and multiply by 0.8. A woman who weighs 135 pounds would do 62 kg x 0.8 and would need 50 grams of protein.

4. Keep a steady blood sugar level by eating every two to three hours

Make sure you keep healthy snacks on hand everywhere you go. If you make sure you have all the right stuff hidden in places like your glove compartment, purse, and office drawers, you will be less tempted to make a trip to the corner store or vending machine.

5.   A crock pot will save you time and hassle during the winter

Soup makes you feel happy and warm and you can fill it with as many alkaline forming veggies as you want. Add in some good for you beans and you will get a good protein boost. Pick broth over a cream-based soup.

6.   Start with green smoothies

If you begin your day with an energizing green smoothie, you will start it off with two to three servings of veggies. A lot of people struggle to eat first thing in the morning, which is when it is the most important. An alkaline smoothie will help to get your motor running and will boost your energy.

If you make sure that you follow the tips in this chapter, you will be well on your way to forming healthy habits and an alkaline diet.

Conclusion

Thank for making it through to the end of *Alkaline Diet*, let's hope it was informative and able to provide you with all of the tools you need to achieve your goals whatever they may be.

With the information that you have, you can now start a successful alkaline diet. Your body works better when it isn't acidic. The alkaline diet ensures that your body works its best. The great thing is, all of the food you can eat is tasty. With the recipes in this book, you won't have to worry about what you are going to fix for dinner. Don't wait any longer. Get started today and see your body change for the better.

CPSIA information can be obtained
at www.ICGtesting.com
Printed in the USA
BVHW050014090421
604476BV00005B/1393